Joanne Prentice, Kit CBx

P9-DBN-363

What people are saying about Dying to Change...

"Katie Jay brings insight, humor, and refreshing honesty to the deeply personal subject of obesity as we witness her amazing life transformation through weight loss surgery. I couldn't put the book down."
— Paula F. Peck, RN, author of *Exodus from Obesity*

"Katie doesn't hold anything back. Her psychological and emotional insights are right on. This book is intense!"
— Patricia Walker, MFT

"*Dying to Change* is full of useful information for people who want an insider's look at weight loss surgery; but more than that, it is full of courage, hope, and inspiration. This is the story of a woman who struggled and triumphed in life despite her numerous challenges."
— Kimberly Martin, WLS patient

Dying to
CHANGE

from the director of the National Association for Weight Loss Surgery

Dying to CHANGE

my really heavy life story

How weight loss
surgery gave me
hope for living...

Katie Jay

Dying to Change: My Really Heavy Life Story by Katie Jay

Published by Pink Sky, Inc. — www.pinkskyinc.com. Available to the trade from all major wholesalers. For information regarding distribution, please contact Pink Sky, Inc. at 1-877-PinkSky or visit www.pinkskyinc.com.

© 2006 by Katie Jay. All rights reserved. No part of this book may be reproduced in any form or by any electronic or mechanical means, including information storage and retrieval systems, without written permission from the publisher, except by a reviewer, who may quote brief passages. The views expressed are those of Katie Jay or Pink Sky, Inc. Although the author and publisher have made every effort to ensure the accuracy and completeness of the information contained in this book, we assume no responsibility for errors, inaccuracies, omissions, or any inconsistencies herein. Any slights to people, places, or organizations are unintentional.

The author and publisher of this book are not engaged in rendering medical advice or services. The information, statements and opinions set forth in and referred to in this book are neither intended nor are implied to be a substitute for professional medical advice. Always seek the advice of your physician or other qualified health care provider prior to starting any new treatment or with any questions you may have regarding a medical condition. Many factors unknown to the author and publisher may affect the applicability of any information, statements and opinions set forth in and referred to in this book to your particular circumstances. You should not act or refrain from acting based upon any information contained in this book without consulting a qualified healthcare professional. If you have or suspect you have a health problem, you should contact your healthcare provider immediately. This book contains general information that is not specific to any individual person. If you have questions after reading this, ask your own physician or healthcare professional or provider. They know you and can best answer your questions. The author and publisher expressly disclaim any liability for loss, damage or injury caused by the contents of this book.

All brand, product, service, and company names are trademarks of their respective holders. Reference to a product, service, or company does not imply recommendation, approval, affiliation, or sponsorship of that product, service, or company by either the author or Pink Sky, Inc.

Cover and interior design by Pneuma Books, LLC. Visit www.pneumabooks.com for more information.

Publisher's Cataloging-in-Publication Data
(Prepared by The Donohue Group, Inc.)

Jay, Katie.
    Dying to change : my really heavy life story : how weight loss
surgery gave me hope for living / Katie Jay.   .

        p. ; cm.
    At head of title: From the director of the National Association for Weight Loss Surgery
    ISBN-13: 978-0-9772289-4-2 (Hardcover)
    ISBN-13: 978-0-9772289-0-4 (pbk.)
    ISBN-10: 0-9772289-4-0 (Hardcover)
    ISBN-10: 0-9772289-0-8 (pbk.)

1. Gastric bypass–Patients–Biography. 2. Gastric bypass–Popular works. 3. Overweight women–United States–Biography. 4. Obesity–Surgery. I. National Association for Weight Loss Surgery. II. Title. III. Title: From the director of the National Association for Weight Loss Surgery.

RD540.5 .J39 2005
616.3/9806   2005907950

Printed and bound in the United States of America
11 10 09 08 07 06   6 5 4 3 2 1

For God, who suffers with us.
To Mike and Barrett, who love me unconditionally.

Table of Contents

Preface

At forty-four years of age, I still found myself cringing every time my mother told me how concerned she was about my weight. What she really meant was *You look like hell. Fat is disgusting. You're disgusting.*

For the first time since young adulthood, my mother and I were living under the same roof. She had been diagnosed with metastasized breast cancer, and my husband, Mike, and I decided to have her come live with us so that we could take care of her. She lived with us for about fourteen months, providing me with an opportunity to get in touch with all of my resentment toward her and about the way she criticized my food choices, eating habits, and weight.

Every evening that she lived with us, she came to the dinner table, picked at her food, and said things to Mike and me like, "Are you going to eat all that?" She would crinkle up her nose and examine every detail of what we put on our plates. She would point out food items or condiments she found repulsive with comments like: "You put catsup on your eggs? That's disgusting!"

I already knew I had issues with my mother, but her year with us made me realize how rebellious I felt around her. I began to line up the napkin holder and any bottles or boxes on the table so that she couldn't see what was on my plate. I didn't plan to do that. I just noticed one evening that I had created a shield around my plate.

I noticed I ate my bowl of ice cream at bedtime with a defiant attitude. Even though Mom wasn't present for those episodes, she was in my head criticizing me with every bite. I told myself I didn't care. I needed the ice cream, because it relieved my stress and made me feel nurtured.

During the year my mom was with us, my son, Barrett, was the most patient, kind, and unselfish boy I have ever known. While Mom was with us, I can't even guess how many times I said to him, "I can't, Barrett, I need to take care of Grandma right now."

After Mom was gone, I wanted to give him my undivided attention. So when my dear friend Pat told me she was taking her two sons to Disney, Barrett and I decided to meet them there. Despite my initial reluctance, it seemed like the perfect opportunity to have some fun with Barrett.

There is no way I could have done Disney walking. I didn't decide to go until a friend suggested I rent a wheelchair. A wheelchair? I had never even considered renting one of those. At first, I was stunned at the suggestion, even though it made sense. My second reaction was relief. I feel sad remembering how relieved I was to surrender to a wheelchair.

The only downside to the wheelchair was that Pat had to push me. She was a great sport about it, but I did have to endure a bit of discussion about why I wasn't walking more. Wouldn't it help me to lose weight? No matter that I did more walking at Disney (even using the wheelchair some of the time) than I had at home in a long, long time. Being so heavy, I had stopped going to the grocery store, rarely ran errands — heck, I couldn't walk half a block without getting major back and foot pain.

At one point, Pat questioned me because I hadn't taken the stairs at a restaurant — I had used the elevator. That woman is so fit and so able, I don't think she realized how hard it was for me to carry around 331 pounds everywhere I went. She felt I was making excuses, I imagine. I felt hurt and ashamed, once again wishing I could be thin for someone who cared about me.

I remember thinking, *I'm not going to lose weight ever again. I just can't. I don't have another try in me.* I don't think I said that to Pat. I just talked about how hard it was to stop overeating and how badly I felt. Honestly, I don't remember exactly what I said. I know I felt ashamed and resigned to my obesity.

Yep. We had one of those dreadful conversations in which the thin person who cares about the obese person wonders aloud why the obese person isn't doing more to remedy the situation. Pat didn't seem to understand why I couldn't lose weight. In that moment, I didn't understand either. I was completely humiliated.

Pat did get me thinking, though. In the days following our Disney trip, I stewed and agonized. Why was it so hard for me to lose weight and keep it off? Then one night I stayed up until 3 A.M. writing in my journal. The writing helped me realize that there was no single reason why I was obese. Yet I prayed to find a solution. I felt stuck. I felt like I couldn't change my situation, nor could I keep on going the way I was going.

The result of all my stewing and writing was that I had an emotional and spiritual breakthrough, and my life course changed dramatically. Thank God. The story in the pages that follow has been gleaned from what turned into a collection of journal entries written during the months leading up to and following my transformational experience — my last hope.

I want people to understand how complex and painful the disease of obesity is. And by telling my story, I want to bring compassion and understanding to people suffering with this devastating problem.

To my obese comrades, I say we are neither worthless nor hopeless — and it's time for the entire medical community to acknowledge what medical professionals like the doctor who suggested weight loss surgery (WLS) to me and my WLS surgeon already know: the truth about obesity and a way to treat it that works pretty damn well.

I want fellow human beings to treat us with respect and compassion. Heck, we need to treat ourselves with respect and compassion. Please don't give up. Have courage.

Simply Complicated

When I had a heart-to-heart talk with my husband, Mike, about having weight loss surgery (WLS), which is also known as gastric bypass, I recalled all the stages and struggles I had been through over the years as I tried to control my weight — albeit unsuccessfully. I now weighed 331 pounds and had type II diabetes and rising blood pressure. I had reached the point where my health and spirit were deteriorating exponentially.

As we discussed my health problems and my hopelessness about solving them, Mike used the phrase *simply complicated* to describe me. He knew the difficult time I had had getting help from doctors who didn't understand me or know how to properly treat obese patients.

My husband asserted that the solution to my health problems was multifaceted — okay, complicated.

Actually, Mike had begun referring to me as *simply complicated* right around the time my mother came to live with us. During the year that I took care of my mother, I was also homeschooling my son, Barrett, and struggling with my own health. I was stressed out, exhausted, and stuffing my emotions with food. I didn't know what to do. It *was* complicated. With such a needy mom, I didn't take the time to go to doctors who wouldn't understand my obesity problem anyway. Being diagnosed as "fat" over and over again was depressing and frustrating, because I knew there had to be more to my solution than diet and exercise.

To add to the challenge, *I* am complicated. Mike said, "Don't worry about it. You've always been complicated," and then he gave me his best impish smile.

Have I? I knew I was deep, too intense (according to my sister, Sarah), sensitive, Mensa-eligible (according to my psychologist), *and* struggling with addiction (recovering alcoholic for twenty-one years). But now, as I talked to my husband about how I could get the help I needed to overcome my weight problem, he used that phrase again — *simply complicated.*

I know some of the reasons I reached the point of being what the doctors call "super morbidly obese," but my obesity did not follow this simple recipe: Take one crazy woman, feed her too much food, stir, and *voila*! My recipe was much more complicated than that. It was more like: Take one extremely sensitive woman; sprinkle in a mixture of genius and intensity; add a pinch each of emotional abuse, tough life circumstances, a dysfunctional family, attention deficit hyperactivity disorder (ADHD), depression, and physical illness; blend while slowly pouring in more alcohol than necessary; and top it off with way too much chocolate.

But that's only half the recipe. The reason I'm obese but not dead is because my recipe also includes creativity, a sense of humor, kindness, compassion, a strong desire to improve myself, willpower, extensive twelve-step training, and a lifelong search for God.

I never felt I had the innate ability to heal myself, so I have prayed and sought help from professional after professional over the years — always trying to find the single answer to my unhappiness. *Maybe it's because of this. Maybe it's because of that,* I would say hopefully, thinking there was a magic key. The professionals and I never found a single answer. In fact, every time we thought we did, we uncovered another problem.

Needless to say, I have baffled many professionals. I am articulate, more self-aware than most, intensely honest, and open to trying almost anything to feel better. (A problem in and of itself!) What frustrated the professionals is that most interventions never really helped. If I was lucky, they worked for a while, but eventually I was back to where I started or worse.

Over the course of twenty years, I've tried family-of-origin therapy, individual therapy (at least five different times), group therapy for overeaters, past-life regression, guided imagery, every twelve-step program known to man, hospitalizations for alcoholism and an eating disorder, and treatment for being the child of an alcoholic. I've tried Weight Watchers, an all-liquid protein diet, and NutriSystem. And that's just a partial list.

The so-called professionals who have helped me the least in my life have been medical doctors. It seems my delicate interplay of emotional and physical problems has, for the most part, bewildered them. You see, I'm no easy-to-swallow smoothie. I'm chunky (pun intended)!

For ten years or so, I had given up on losing weight — given up on myself. I decided I had tried everything, no one was offering much help, and there was nothing anyone could do. I was doomed to a life of pain and illness. *Doomed.*

Despite all the bad experiences I had had with doctors, I mustered up the courage to make an appointment with a newly discovered, holistic physician. I went in to see this general practitioner (GP) soon after my mother died. I was finally free to take care of myself. As I sat in the doctor's office describing my situation, I felt vulnerable and profoundly sad.

I was so obese my health had begun to seriously fail. The examination gown was way too small, and I was embarrassed that I might tip over the examination table when I hoisted myself onto it. My mother had just died in my home, and Mike's mom had also recently died. (He had spent the last year traveling seven hours back and forth every other weekend to help care for her.) I was grieving the loss of my health too. Desperate to feel better, I wanted my new doctor to finally unlock the mystery of my obesity and help me get my health back.

Every doctor up to this point had ordered, "Lose weight. Go home, eat right, and exercise." *What a concept! And so simple. Why hadn't I thought of it?* I told my GP that research had shown that anywhere from 95 to 98 percent of people who diet gain all the weight back, plus some. I told her I was scared to get any larger than I was now. As we reviewed all my health problems, I told her how hard it had been to take care of myself *and* my challenging family. My GP said, "You might want to get some therapy." *Great idea! I hadn't thought of that before either.*

The decision to see my GP was the beginning of a new chapter in my life. I had read an article in *The Washington Post* that gave me some new ideas about how obese people should approach medical doctors. The article suggested that we ask our doctors to treat us the same as they would a thin patient. Ask them to do the same lab tests they would do on a thin patient and to treat our illnesses aggressively to minimize the damage our weight causes. Tell them not to assume when they look at us that we don't care about our health.

It took courage, but I did it — I called the doctors on this age-old prejudice. To my surprise, my GP, and the specialists she referred me to, ultimately took me seriously and responded to my demands. And that has made all the difference.

I began to accept that I was a complicated, nontraditional patient. And, more importantly, I didn't allow my shame to stop me from asking for what I needed. I stopped requiring myself to be perfect. I finally realized that I didn't need to be perfect to deserve help.

Maybe you know people who are perfect. They begin as well-behaved children and are positive, goal-oriented adolescents. They succeed in all subjects and sports. They get into the best universities and get scholarships. They find good jobs, pick good mates, and have wonderful friends. Their kids are chips off the old block. They come from good families. They are beautiful. They don't have bad breath. They are thin. They are addiction-free. They can stop after one piece of chocolate. They have no spiritual confusion or doubts. They are prosperous. And they have great singing voices.

Growing up, I thought I was supposed to be perfect. I was criticized so much, and I couldn't forgive myself for any aspect of my life that deviated from my ideal of perfection. I began a lifelong habit of monitoring everything I said, did, and was. The self-consciousness put a damper on so much. I didn't have free abandon. I never have.

Okay, I had it once. It was right after I met and fell in love with my husband. He was an accomplished swimmer, and his high school coach had taught him how to meditate to prepare for swim meets. I had never been in a meditative state, and I wanted him to help me get into one. He had me lie down; close my eyes; and breathe long, slow breaths. I felt as happy as a little girl whose father was giving her his rare, undivided attention.

Mike said gently, "Deep breaths, Kitten [his nickname for me]. Deep and free."

I knew he was looking at me, and under normal circumstances I would have been too self-conscious to tolerate that (as it was, I had to dismiss thoughts about him noticing my ugly eyebrows). But because we were newly in love, I felt safer with Mike than I ever had with anyone. I began to giggle, and as I started to rein in my laughter and cover my face (my eyebrows), Mike gently moved my hands and whispered, "Deep and free. Let yourself laugh if that's what you feel." So I just giggled away, with my face uncovered, and let Mike look at me. I had a fleeting sense of euphoria, but it was too difficult to allow this feeling of exposure to continue for long. The fact that I remember this experience so vividly shows me how profoundly self-conscious I've been nearly all my life. I rarely let my guard down and never all the way.

Needy or Neglected?

I was born complicated. I have always had an energy and passion that overwhelmed those around me. I had needs it seemed few others had. My dad must have said to me a thousand times, "Katie, the game is over." But I always wanted to keep playing.

I was philosophical at a very young age and thus periodically experienced an existential depression that must have floored my family. And I was needy. I wanted more than the world could possibly give me: more nurturing, more opportunity, more excitement, more forgiveness, more understanding, more love, more chocolate.

So I nurtured myself with food in a society that encouraged that behavior. I hid food under my mattress, ate all the candy bars I was supposed to be selling for school, stole candy from the market down the street, and ate Sarah's snack cakes. I was passionate about food, and now I realize that I was craving its calming, comforting effects.

People walking down the street now feel entitled to call me fat. But day after day, year after year, I have been told by commercials and by friends that I deserve to indulge in all kinds of edible treats (a birthday cake, for example). Do I? It's complicated.

Some mean boys at the country club we belonged to called me tank when I hit puberty. TANK YOU VERY MUCH, BOYS. Apparently, I was a tank with attractive, large breasts. No one seemed to mind the breasts. In fact, males were always finding ways to ogle and touch them.

My boss at the hotel where I worked as a front desk clerk while I was in college would approach me in the morning and pull open the front of my blazer (I had a blouse on underneath). Then this pervert would inhale deeply while looking at my chest, and he'd shake his head and drawl, "Mmm, mmm, mmmmm-mmm, very nice."

My round hips and large legs, however, were cause for criticism by some. That's where the tank part came in. This mixed attention was confusing to me. I didn't know if I was attractive or despicable. When I got positive male attention, I didn't know if a boy liked me for my personality or if he just wanted sex. I'm sure both were the case at times, but it was complicated, especially after my dad left (more about that later).

If my life was a dinner party, and the family I grew up with was seated at the table, the seating chart would be complicated, of course.

At the head of the table would sit my inattentive and complicated father. (The man my mother, who was his first wife, loved until the day she died.) Sitting securely next to my father on the same chair would be my stepmother. Sitting on the floor next to her with arms wrapped around her leg and begging for attention would be my sweet stepbrother. (My peeved father would be trying to kick him away.) Far on the other end of the table would sit my fearful, self-absorbed mother, who was almost consumed by self-loathing. My two, sharp, long-lived grandmothers would sit on opposite sides of the table. (They were as different as night and day.) Their husbands (my grandfathers) were a couple of abusive alcoholics and were both dead before I was out of elementary school. They would never be allowed to sit at our family table, if I had my way. Sarah would sit between my mother and me, and I would sit between my father and Sarah.

Of course, these people would never have been at a table together in real life. My mother never even met my stepmother in the twenty-six years my dad was married to her. I don't think either woman wanted to meet. Today, my mother, grandmothers, and stepmother are gone.

I have loved and do love all the people at my table deeply. We have all hurt each other at times, but we have laughed with each other as well. Like most families, we have cried together and shared great joys. Despite some difficult times in my family, I wouldn't change it for anything. I love my family, but I have to be honest in my story. I don't intend to hurt feelings or represent anyone as anything but human and worthy of respect and forgiveness, just like me.

I wish we all *could* sit at a dinner table together.

I still can't believe my mother has "left the table." She was another complicated one. (She had been an abused child, she was a depressive, and she loved to drink.) She was diagnosed with breast cancer about six years ago after she'd been showing symptoms for way too long. I don't know why she didn't go to the doctor sooner. I think in some ways she had given up.

Mom had a mastectomy after her initial diagnosis but refused radiation and chemotherapy. She said she didn't want to suffer the discomfort of those treatments. Having watched my mother-in-law battle cancer until the end, I can't say my mom made a bad decision. It just hurt that she didn't want to fight and that she didn't want to live a long time. She had watched her mother die miserably in her early ninties, and my mom didn't want that ending.

When Mom's cancer returned five years later, she tried an oral medication but once again refused chemotherapy. She basically decided that she would let the cancer run its course.

We brought Mom to live with us for the last year of her life. She did not spend the year feeling self-pity, nor, to my surprise, was she horribly depressed. She spent the year telling the hospice people she couldn't believe she had cancer, because she felt pretty good. What a godsend that was. (Personally, I think she felt good because we had reduced her alcohol intake, which probably had been irritating her liver — the place to which her cancer had metastasized.)

Her last words were to a beloved friend who was trying to make sure my mom was comfortable. By this time, Mom was mostly non-communicative. She was lying in bed with her eyes closed, only stirring when a noise sounded and even then not opening her eyes.

Mom's friend of more than forty years, who also happens to be a nurse, asked, "Jane, do you want me to turn you on your side?"

I noticed the almost imperceptible shake of Mom's head. I had learned to read her signals in our last year together.

"I think she's okay," I volunteered.

"Jane? Why don't I turn you on your side for a bit." Mom's friend wanted so badly to do *something*.

"She's okay," I said, detecting a slight frown on Mom's face every time her friend asked the question.

"Well, I want her to be comfortable. Do you want to be on your side, Jane?"

My mom finally responded with her blunt humor, "If you ask me that one more time, I'm going to hit you."

Her last words. We all laughed, and Mom slipped back into her restful state. She wanted to go, despite her loving family. She *wanted* to go. Deep down, I fear maybe we weren't worth staying for.

Even during her final days, my mother was bothered by my weight. I think she wanted me to take care of myself, but she was very demanding during our year together. This made it hard for me to take time for myself. That was her way. The year was about her, and she came in and took charge, not even realizing she was doing it.

Our relationship was complicated. I was an exemplary care-taker. And she, Sarah, and I knew my home was the best place for Mom to be. I am the nurturing one in the family. (At the same time, Sarah took Mom home to spend the night every chance she got and was in and out of our house constantly — what a relief!)

Despite her desire to live with me, Mom was critical of how I looked and lived. Of course, that's how I found myself hiding my dinner plate. She would sit at the table with us and eat about one-fifth what we did. She had the declining appetite that comes with cancer.

"Are you going to eat all that?" she'd ask my husband. I hated that. He hated that. She continued, "Oooooo, are you eating that too, Katie? How can you all eat so much?" Oh, how I hated Mom's dinnertime commentary.

I have in my heart endless hurts due to the thoughtless, and sometimes cruel, things my mother said to me over the years — things like, "You have such a pretty face." My mother used to say that to me all the time. What a shame I was so fat. She found my body detestable. I think it was her own self-loathing, in part, that made her so uncomfortable with my imperfections.

There is one time, however, that burns in my memory and hurts like hell, even as I write this. Barrett's delivery by cesarean left me with a scar and a postoperative infection on the incision line. I was supposed to change the dressing a couple of times a day, but I couldn't see the incision line due to my recent pregnancy and ensuing roundness. Isn't that somewhat common?

So I asked my mom to help me change the dressing, but when I pulled down the covers and displayed the wound area, my mother's face contorted in disgust. She said, "Will that stomach ever go away?"

My face must have flushed with shock; I held my breath the way you do when you've been punched in the stomach. How could I possibly have thought my mother was the right person to ask for help? There's nothing quite like being kicked by your mother when you're down. And I was down. I had postpartum depression, a husband who was working full-time and attending graduate school... and a colicky baby. Those were tough times, made exceedingly more so by my mother's harsh judgment and lack of compassion.

The first time I was called fat, I was in fifth grade. I was having trouble finding something to wear, and the hot pants and jacket made out of quilted brown material — decorated with pink flowers no less — did not look good. (I'm not sure they would have looked good on anyone.) I was modeling the outfit for my dad. I think I was frustrated that the outfit did not fit comfortably, I'm not sure. But I do remember my dad saying, "Kate, you're fat!"

There. That was it — the first time I realized my physical appearance was not acceptable. Heck, I didn't know it at the time, but I was about to get my first period. I was developing breasts early. I was curvy. I was disgusting to my family.

Sarah used to complain that I was too heavy when we horsed around in the front yard. I was stronger than her. Then my mother started hiding sweet treats from me. Hey, I ate them because they were there and they tasted good. But I felt singled out, and I imagined I was the one family member who could not have sweets at will.

Then Mom started buying me diet soft drinks. She put me on a protein diet when I was eleven years old, right after my dad told me I was fat.

Interestingly, years later I looked at my childhood pictures with a therapist and she teared up, which really surprised me. "You were a beautiful young woman," she said softly. "You were not a particularly fat child. You were not skinny, but you were not abnormally overweight for a girl beginning puberty."

If I had heard that same message from my family when I was growing up, I can only imagine how my life might have been different.

3

Doctors Behaving Badly

The Fools Hall of Fame in my life is crowded. Of course, I'm in it, but it irks me that so many of my physicians and nurses are in it too. I have not been silent about my condition. I have articulated well that I have tried everything I can think of and have not been able to resolve my weight problem to nearly every doctor I've seen. I gave up sugar and white flour for more than a year. I tried a liquid protein diet with great success, only to gain the weight back. I attended support groups for compulsive overeaters for a long, long time and did what I was told.

Still, I'm perceived as fat and lazy. I have more willpower than most people I know. It's not a willpower problem. That has been scientifically proven, yet many doctors and the general public don't seem to get it.

Would a smoker who has lung cancer choose the treatment that is 2–5 percent effective or the one that is 70 percent effective? That is why I've decided to have WLS. It's not that I can't lose the weight; it's knowing that 95 percent of people who lose weight don't keep it off. A much higher percentage of WLS recipients keep their weight off. So, why wouldn't I choose this option with the better outcome percentages?

"Weight loss surgery is so drastic!" I hear it all the time. And every time I think, *Why am I judged for not choosing the 2–5 percent solution? Why does the media portray WLS as so incredibly dangerous? Why is WLS coverage so biased that people jump to the wrong conclusion?*

I admit that when I first learned about WLS, I didn't even give it consideration. I knew Carnie Wilson was having it, and I was surprised that she was broadcasting it live on the Internet. I didn't think the topic was relevant to my situation. A few years later, when I learned that my roommate from an inpatient eating disorder treatment program had had WLS, I still didn't perceive it as an option for myself.

She is truly hopeless, I thought but not in a negative way. I just didn't think I was that bad off.

Before my inpatient treatment, I had a bout of chronic fatigue accompanied by severe body and joint pain. It lasted about a year and I treated it aggressively because my doctors wouldn't. They only diagnosed me as fat. One doctor rolled her eyes at me. Another called me a hypochondriac. And another had a mean nurse who, after making me wait well over an hour for a fasting blood test, claimed in a condescending voice that doing the blood work was a courtesy. Is that why I had to make an appointment and pay a fee? A courtesy? In retrospect, I wonder if the nurse felt it was somehow okay to speak rudely to a fat person. That's what a wafer-thin friend of mine suspected.

This friend has always had every ache and pain scrutinized by every physician she has ever gone to as if it could be a *very serious problem.* When she was in her mid-thirties, she complained of slight chest pain and was sent home with a portable heart monitor to wear for the weekend. I've complained of chest pain several times in the past, but I've never been sent home on a monitor. She also was tested for Lyme Disease and Epstein-Barr virus when she felt fatigued.

I complained of fatigue to Dr. Eye Roller, and she prescribed NOTHING. Then I went to an infectious disease doctor, who refused to do any testing. To my astonishment, he said I did not have any symptoms that concerned him. Finally, I went to an alternative physician (paid out of pocket, of course), who did the blood work and found parasitic and bacterial infections.

After I used the alternative antibiotic treatments and antiparasitic herbs, I was still fat, but I was so much happier — and much livelier. My blood sugar readings dropped significantly for a while following these treatments as well. Hmmm. That should be researched, but will doctors take the time to do that research? Probably not. I was so relieved to feel better — much less joint pain, no fatigue. Amazing. Apparently, the malady had not been directly related to my weight. It was prejudice, pure prejudice.

I went to hear a speaker share her story about gastric bypass surgery, and she said that once she made the decision to have the surgery, she felt hope for the first time in many years. I feel the same way now. I can't imagine why such an important medical tool was never mentioned to me by the many doctors I have seen. It is one thing to be aware of a treatment; it's quite another to have your doctor tell you that you need it and should pursue it. My insurance company will probably save money in the long run if I get the surgery, yet it presents hoop after hoop after hoop, obstacle after obstacle. You get the picture.

One hoop is a psychological evaluation. When was the last time a heart surgery candidate or cancer patient underwent a psychiatric evaluation before surgery? I am emotionally healthier and more self-aware than most people I know. I am so frustrated by the types of questions I have had to answer for the psychologist. Do I hear voices? (If so, would I deserve to die of morbid obesity? Do schizophrenics get treatment for cancer and heart disease?) Do I see things that aren't there? (Should that matter?) Do I believe it's okay to steal? Do I (and I'm not kidding here, this was on the questionnaire) think I'd make a good sports reporter?

What does my psychological state have to do with treating my type II diabetes, arthritis, gastro-esophageal reflux disease, autoimmune thyroid condition, and obesity — to name a few of my health problems? Do lung cancer patients who smoke have to have a psychological evaluation before they have part of a lung removed or receive chemotherapy? Of course not. Hating fat people is one of the last prejudices that is socially acceptable in our country.

Fools do make us suffer, don't they?

When I read the story of Job, I was shocked to learn it was a sin to blame God for troubles he allowed to come into our lives — not troubles we have brought on ourselves, but troubles He has allowed to occur. In light of that realization, clearly I couldn't blame God for my problems. But, is he my solution?

God decided to test Job by allowing Satan, the accuser, to nearly ruin Job's life. God wanted to prove Job's devotion. I have to wonder, though, what was the purpose of destroying Job's first set of children? Were they blasphemous? Did God see no hope in them? Were they not worthy of his love and mercy? Were they fat?

I imagine we are not supposed to value this life too much, knowing God can take us whenever he wants. We are supposed to be comforted by the assurance of a hereafter. I secretly fear that God views me in the same light as Job's original children, in which case I'm dust.

Relying on God, the mysterious, can be hard. Some of us suffer immeasurably as we attempt to clear our God-approved hurdles. Some of us, the complicated ones, have so many hurdles it seems ridiculous. What is God's purpose in *that*?

Some believers say the hurdles make us rely on God, draw us to him. That is one possibility. Some of us, however, become confused. If God is Love, what was he thinking when he squashed Job's children like bugs? He was calling them home, but is it really a sin to blame God for allowing them to be pawns in a game that didn't include peace on Earth for them?

My desire for life on Earth is strong. I want to live. Don't most of us? Why does God give us a strong will to live and then force us to grapple endlessly with our doom? I guess God has a purpose for each person's suffering. We can't ever know if we've had our share, because, praise God, we might have more at any moment. It's a confusing mix of temptation, thanks be to God, and suffering, thanks be to God. Okay, I'm angry at God. I admit it. I don't get what his plan is for me. I mean, is he FOR ME or am I a pawn too? (Maybe I should be focusing on being FOR HIM.)

Despite my confusion, I've decided to put my recovery in God's hands. Does he want me to recover? I want to believe he does, but I feel overwhelmed by the challenge of stepping away from a long-ingrained lifestyle of sugar gobbling and junk-food fanaticism. Only time will tell. I believe God put the notion of WLS in my life. I certainly didn't go looking for that particular solution. Is the lesson to be learned from Job that we can make God-fearing, sinless choices in our lives (like Job) and still be put through the wringer? I hope the wringer is behind me.

Don't let the low-carb products fool you. Americans love to eat sugar and junk food — and still do it all the time. I can't seem to stop eating the things I think I won't be able to have once I have WLS. Today it was a fried egg sandwich. Actually, I'm not sure I'll have to avoid fried egg sandwiches after the surgery, but I suspect they won't be the number one meal recommendation.

I know what it's like to have to avoid certain foods. Part of the reason I put off dieting again is that it's so hard to be confronted day after day with food items I cannot or should not eat. For more than a year, I took "appropriate" food with me everywhere I went — even to business luncheons, luncheons at which cheesecake was served. Boy, did I get some strange looks. It was hard to watch others eat things I knew I shouldn't. Considering that only 2–5 percent of dieters keep their weight off, it's easy to see that deprivation is a big issue. Self-denial is not a popular part of our fast-food, credit-card culture.

Mike and I recently decided to put Barrett in school for the last couple months of the school year because of my poor health and other things. Barrett's school smells like sugar. I noticed it when I went to pick him up. I had always known it subconsciously, but then it hit me like a ton of sugar cane. It was not just a sugar odor but a distinct cookie smell. I asked about it. I was told that cookie parties are the reward for good behavior at the school. Cookie parties? Oh my goodness. It must be an evil plot to feed our children mass quantities of sugar, so that they will crave mass quantities of sugar, so they will buy mass quantities of sugar products when they start to spend their own money. And then we'll criticize them for getting fat.

Don't we Americans enjoy that? We like to create movie stars and then see them fall. Many of our politicians start out idealists and then are seduced by fame and power, only to fall. Why not turn our sweets-loving children into sugar addicts?

What are we doing to our children? I want to have a sugar-free son. I don't want him to develop a cycle like the one I developed. My family denied me treats, so I began to treat myself in secret. I don't want that for Barrett. Ever since he was little, I have served him balanced meals and very small portions of sweets on occasion. I wanted him to have the treats but also to understand their appropriate place in his diet. Well, the cookie parties undermine that. So do the school candy sales, the birthday cakes, and the TV commercials. (We didn't even let our son watch anything but PBS until he was ten years old, in part so that he would not be exposed to the commercials.)

What a disappointment that Barrett's new school classifies cookie parties as a reward. Nice lesson.

I'm Not the Only One — Am I?

When I got sober in 1983, my family and some of my friends accused me of using my newfound knowledge about alcoholism to diagnose some of them as alcoholics. My mother certainly blacked out a lot in her later years. I wanted so badly to assimilate them into my life, to feel like they understood me. To this day I'm not sure if they were right, or if I was.

As I approach WLS, I think about my obese friends and wonder if any of them will follow the path I am choosing. One friend was very upset when she heard I was considering the surgery. She said, "What would happen if you started walking ten minutes a day? What would happen then?" Of course, I know what would happen. I'd change for a while and then revert back to my old ways. Won't work. Been there, done that.

I have to think through and plan for how I will act and react after I have the surgery, because I will still be a food-loving choco-holic. I know down to my core that I will have to abstain from sweets and high-fat foods. I know I will have to eat a restricted quantity. I guarantee it will be hard at times to resist temptation. So, what will be different? Why is the success rate so much higher for obese people who have WLS as opposed to those who diet?

I'm told that despite psychological cravings for one's old favorites, the surgery curbs the appetite, and frankly, you just can't fit in as much food without throwing up. I would have to really work at blowing the success of the surgery. It can be done, however, which is why I am going to take full advantage of the aftercare program my surgeon offers. The aftercare program is essential.

Here are all the things I have heard are associated with success:

1. Following the aftercare program
2. Drinking water (but not fifteen to thirty minutes before or at least thirty minutes after a meal)
3. Eating protein first
4. Exercising
5. Attending a support group
6. Identifying trigger foods — while avoiding sweets, high-fat foods, refined carbs, and snacking
7. Taking the necessary vitamins and supplements
8. Taking personal responsibility for your weight

WLS requires a lifelong commitment to self-care and medical man-agement. I am ready to do that. I am afraid, though, because I know that making healthy food choices and not overeating get harder once one is well on the way to recovering from surgery. A man in the support group meeting said that when you start to get hungry again and can handle a certain amount of food you become more vulnerable to making unhealthy choices.

I am going to use my twelve-step training for those situations. The twelve-step programs taught me to measure my decisions about what to do in life (at any level of decision — from what to eat to what career I choose) by asking myself one question: Is this choice going to bring me closer to the old patterns of behavior or further away?

Now I will have to ask myself that question regarding my food choices. When I am invited to a friend's house who I know pushes desserts, I must ask myself, "Will going to Mary Lou's bring me closer to blowing my recovery or further away?" I must ask myself on my birthday, "Will having a party with cake bring me closer to sneak eating or further away?" Or, if I am going on vacation, "Will this vacation bring me closer to overeating or further away?" Or, when I need to cook for Barrett, "Will making this mac and cheese bring me closer to blowing my WLS surgery or further away?"

If any of my answers to these questions is *closer,* then I can't do it. I have to be willing to put myself first. You may ask, "What kind of mother wouldn't make food for her child?" Well, my child is eleven years old. And he'd rather have me around to read to him and play games with him — to someday meet his wife and enjoy his kids. He wants to go running with me. He doesn't want to deal with questions and insults from people about his humongous mother. I don't have to feel guilty about choosing to parent differently so that I can save myself and be there for him.

I got the approval letter from my insurance company yesterday. It is official. I am going through with the surgery. I am elated and relieved. I know it won't be all daisies and buttercups, but this budding feeling of hope is taking over. Today when I dropped off my son at school, the teacher asked me if I was interested in working at the school next year (they need a literature lady). Knowing that I will have had the surgery by then, I actually thought, *Hey! That would be fun.* I wonder how many more things will seem fun as I imagine myself carrying around so much less weight. Imagine the implications in my bedroom, at dances, on walks around the neighborhood, on vacations, while cleaning my house (okay, maybe my weight isn't the only reason I dread this activity).

Weight is an unrelenting burden. I carry around this big hulk all day, every day, and it is exhausting and sometimes humiliating. When I'm with most people, I try to pretend it doesn't affect me, but I'm probably not very successful at convincing them. My disability is obvious. I get winded so easily and I can't lift much. It's the pits.

I do have fears about the surgery — even though my chances of living a happy, healthy life are much better with the surgery than without. My GP told me the odds are much worse for me if I don't have the surgery (which makes me wonder why she wasn't the one to recommend it), because my diabetes is getting worse, my arthritis is getting worse, my back has begun to hurt, and my weight works against me. When you get this big, your body has a tougher time losing weight, even if you don't eat huge quantities of food. I didn't know that until recently.

When I hear people talking negatively about the procedure or saying it is too dangerous, I realize what denial we all are in. The truth is, I'm a ticking time bomb right now. This surgery is no more dangerous than many common surgeries. The key is to use a highly experienced surgeon who has specialized in gastric bypass for many years. And I am doing that. I wish the surgery had been recommended to me five years ago. I have missed out on so much.

The Bible says the sins of the father are visited upon the son, and I know what that means. In past generations, my family has had challenges and made choices that I am paying for right now. Whew! What a debt I owe.

There is a long history of child abuse, alcoholism, drug addiction, obesity, insanity, and genius in my family. One of the saddest stories I have been told is about a great uncle who died of alcoholism in his mid-forties. My grandmother sat weeping at his bedside as he confessed to her that he had tried everything and just could not stop drinking. He even tried the barbaric treatment of being wrapped in alcohol-soaked rags and forced to drink alcohol until he was extremely sick. (I admit it, I'm imagining swimming in a vat of chocolate right now...) It's called aversion therapy. And it didn't work. I don't know what else he tried, but his struggle ended when he died in that hospital, leaving a wife and five children behind.

I'm sure my grandmother was devastated. I'm sure her brother's death brought up the old feelings of loss concerning their father's death. They lost their father when they were around five years old. He was a drinker who had been out doing what he did best with a friend one evening. Apparently, they were walking home on the train tracks when they were mowed down by the

"2:16 to St. Louis." Grandma's only memory of him was being sat on a fence post so that he could tie her shoes.

Grandma went on to marry an abusive alcoholic, who my mom said peeped at her through her bedroom keyhole while she changed clothes — and worse. Grandma stayed married to him and took care of him until the day he died (younger than necessary from alcoholism, among other things). Grandma relieved her stress by eating and was overweight most of her life. She had a flare of the family genius though. She chose not to drink alcohol, and she got a master's degree while raising my mother in the 1940s. She was an amazingly strong person who managed to find success in life despite her circumstances and foibles. I loved her dearly.

I like to think I take after that grandmother, having a blend of those flaws and that enormous strength. While I didn't avoid alcohol (I started to drink at age thirteen to numb the deep sadness of my parents' divorce), I did manage to quit drinking at age twenty-three, and I have been sober for more than twenty years. And let me tell you, not drinking was a full-time job for a long time. It was damn hard. It took a lot of work, a lot of willpower, and a lot of help from other people and my higher power. Sadly, I have also used food to manage my intense emotions over the years, so I developed an addiction to that too.

I suffered the extreme hardship of parental divorce (don't kid yourself — kids may be resilient but divorce leaves scars), but I have built a strong marriage for myself with the help of an open mind and lots of therapy. Then came the years of multiple miscarriages (like my mother and grandmother), the birth of a child, and then postpartum depression. Depression. Another family legacy.

5

The Story

veryone in my family of origin has struggled with depression at some point in their lives. Some of this depression was situational. (If your father left your family when you were thirteen, you'd probably feel depressed too.)

Okay, I realize now that I have to tell *the story*. I always wind up in this spot, no matter where I'm attempting to go, so I may as well get it over with. What is *it?* The account of my parents' divorce and the ensuing agony.

I grew up in what was a pretty typical family. My father was a government employee who transferred to the private sector when Nixon won the presidency. Dad became vice president of a research and development organization. I'm sure his salary went up quite a bit. I know we started to take much nicer vacations. I'm sure my mother felt proud of him and happy to have financial success (both my parents grew up in poverty).

But I think leaving the government was a disappointment for Dad. He had relished a job that made a contribution to the well-being of people, and he was a proud Democrat who enjoyed turning political ideals into reality. He was a smart man, at times stern, and at times quite humorous. He was intellectually curious and great with his hands. He was always involved in a project.

My mother was a typical housewife. She took Valium (just a lit-tle), smoked cigarettes, and hosted great parties. She had the slightly plump look of a satisfied, at-home mother of two children. She played tennis at the country club, served as president of the PTA, and was a great conversationalist. I remember her taking Spanish classes at the local college, which bothered Dad a bit, she claimed. She didn't think he wanted her to go to college.

By the early seventies, however, Dad was completely dissatisfied with my mother, and none of us knew it — not even Mom. For her, it might have been denial, but for me it was blissful ignorance. Every evening, my dad would come home from work, and the two of them would sit down and have a martini together before dinner. Sometimes Dad had a beer, but they rarely got even tipsy — and then, only at parties.

My childhood had some fun highlights. I remember clearly when our cat Gypsy had kittens, because Sarah and I were at swim team practice and Dad came to pick us up early. When we excit-edly inquired about why he was picking us up early, he simply meowed at us, which totally tickled me. That was the fun side of my dad.

I remember having insomnia. I would be awake late into the night (balancing my pillow on my feet like a circus performer or playing with my stuffed puppy Snicklefritz), and I can remember getting lonely and going into my parents' room to my dad's side of the bed. (Mom was done with me by this time of day.)

I would whisper, "Daddy. Daaaaaddy. I can't sleep."

"Crawl in," he'd gently growl.

I would then snuggle in next to him and put my head on his arm, using it as a pillow. There is no place I enjoyed visiting more in my childhood. I loved the feeling of being close to my dad. I loved the sound of his voice. I would lie there as long as I could and pretend to go to sleep. After a while, Dad would pick me up and carry me back to my bed. He'd tuck me in, kiss me good night, and I would fall blissfully asleep. Boy, were those the good old days.

My parents never fought. I never heard my dad raise his voice. Every once in a while, Mom would be in the kitchen cooking, and we'd hear a few cupboards close a little harder than normal. She'd slam around a while, but nothing ever came of it. No resentments were voiced; no apparent, lingering anger expressed. I thought my parents were happy together.

I loved to watch them dress up for parties. They seemed to have so much fun — Mom, with her teardrop rhinestone earrings and evening gowns, Dad in a tux or sleek suit. Whenever they got dressed up like that to go out, we always took a picture. They always smiled so big. I thought they were beautiful. Happy. How would I know my dad wasn't sexually satisfied? How would I know he regretted having married a woman who wasn't as smart as he? How would I know he didn't feel needed? That he didn't feel enough admiration from us? I can't imagine what we could have done differently.

Notice, I said *we.* Yes, my parents' divorce felt like my dad was leaving me and Sarah too, not just my mom. That's because that is what happened. Dad did not love me enough to stay. No matter what other reasons he had for leaving, I was not worth staying for.

He justified later, "You all didn't need me anymore."

I was thirteen when he left. Why didn't he know thirteen-year-olds *do* need fathers?

When Dad left, I was a freshman in high school. I had gone on my second diet and was as svelte and nubile as any pretty young teen. I was selected for the freshman cheerleading squad and felt, for the first time in my life, like I had achieved something really wonderful. I was full of myself and having fun, and Dad thought I didn't need him any more. He couldn't have been more wrong.

He thought Mom didn't need him and that Sarah didn't need him, either. Sarah was muddling through her sophomore year of high school (not at all pleased I was a cheerleader), and I'm sure had no need for Dad.

That was why he thought it was okay that he left. And Dad expected us to understand that and act maturely about the whole thing — and to be kind to and interested in his vivacious new girl-friend immediately. That's what mature and thoughtful children *do.* (Actually, I grew to love my stepmother over time — but I didn't feel that way when Dad left.)

Here's what happened. This is the part that tears me up inside. Mom, Sarah, and I were so naive, so vulnerable, just *so* clueless. We had all worshiped my father. All of us. He had been the king of the castle, our leader, the person whose attention made us feel worthy and loved.

Sometimes Dad went away on business. In November of 1973, he did just that a few days before Thanksgiving. He was supposed to return home on Thanksgiving Eve. I must have gone to bed with the excitement of knowing Dad would be home later that evening. I woke up Thanksgiving morning and remember feeling giddy, wanting to go in and tickle Dad awake. I think Sarah was with me as we burst into my parents' bedroom, but Dad wasn't there.

So we scurried excitedly to the kitchen. No Dad. We found my mother alone, sitting in her chair with her head down, shoulders hunched, holding a lit cigarette with long ashes. She looked awful.

"Where's Dad?" we chimed before really noticing Mom's sad state.

Mom looked up at us despondently with tears in her eyes. "He's not here. He's never coming home."

I felt like I had been hit in the stomach. I thought Dad was dead, and I began to cry. Sarah assumed a quiet authority and asked, "What happened?"

"Your father's never coming home. He's left us."

What she was saying didn't make sense to me. He wasn't dead? That would be the only reason he'd leave us, wouldn't it? LEAVE US? I was shocked. I continued to sob, but now I felt confusion along with the sadness.

Sarah didn't cry then. She immediately took charge and comforted Mom and me. I don't remember much of our conversation really. Somehow, Mom told us that Dad had lied about going on the business trip and that he'd left us for another woman.

Eventually, we decided we would go ahead with our Thanksgiving dinner with one empty chair at the table.

Sarah put Mom and me to work. I think she had me making the stuffing and Mom was to get the bird ready. Once she had Mom and me busy — still sniffling but focused on making the meal, Sarah — my mature, composed, older sister — announced she was going to go take a shower.

We heard her walk down the hall with purpose, go into the bathroom, shut the door, and turn on the shower. And then, we heard loud, agonizing sobs. I remember Mom and I laughing in surprise, for just a moment.

Mom told us we could not tell anyone Dad had left. So Sarah and I decided we would each tell one friend. My friend didn't believe me when I told her. Nancy and I met at Fort Willard, a woodsy island in the middle of our neighborhood, and we walked from there to her house. I remember going into her backyard to do cartwheels.

"Nancy, guess what?"

"What?" she paused with her hands in the air.

"My dad left."

"Bull, Katie. He did not!" She cartwheeled away from me.

"Uh huh!" I yelled, cartwheeling toward her.

"He did not," she insisted, cartwheeling away again.

"He did too, Nancy. I'm not kidding," I stopped suddenly and stood motionless.

Then I was yelling and crying at the same time, "HE LEFT US!"

"What?" She looked shocked.

I think my parents' divorce surprised a lot of people. I was so overwhelmed with sadness I could barely function. I can remember friends telling me they were sick of hearing me cry all the time. I'm sure the lack of emotional support from my parents contributed to my deep and unyielding sorrow.

In Spanish class, sometime in the weeks that followed, the teacher asked us — in Spanish, of course: "What time does your father come home from work?"

"He doesn't come home from work anymore," I teared up in front of the class when it was my turn to answer. "He left us." I remember leaving the classroom at this point in shame and tears. No one, not even the teacher, came after me.

Years later, I sat with my dad at a restaurant in Oregon. (I had flown out to be with him when my stepmother was dying.) The hospice aide had offered to stay with her while Dad and I went to a steakhouse in a nearby city. Dad had one too many martinis that night, which was understandable. We talked about a lot of things that evening. At one point, our conversation drifted to those awful years in my late teens and early twenties when I was frighteningly messed up by grief and had sunk into alcoholism.

"I know we almost lost you during that time, Kate," my dad said, acknowledging how difficult the divorce had been on me and how crazy and self-destructive I got.

"I know we almost lost you," Dad repeated, "but I wouldn't have done anything differently."

This might surprise some people — despite past suicidal feelings and a whole lot of sadness and loss in my life, I have lived what I consider to be a happy and satisfying life overall. Thankfully, my love of life and my sense of humor have won out over my depression time and time again. I don't know why. So many don't make it. There have been countless times when I have felt scared, sad, and overwhelmed. Yet somehow I know that my life — even as an obese, diseased, depressed woman — is charmed. That must be a family trait too. Damn. The book of Job taught me I can't blame God, and now I realize I can't blame my family either! I see my pathetic pointer finger wagging at God and my family, while I see the rest of my fingers pointing back at me. Damn.

The roots of my depression run deeper than any one situation. I am guessing I was predisposed to depression (I'm not blaming anyone), and then as my life got more and more stressful, my depression grew from a sapling into a large, shady weeping willow tree. But the roots didn't choke the life out of me. And now I have an opportunity to cut off some old branches and have some new growth, through WLS — and sheer determination. Oh yeah, and antidepressant medication — have you been avoiding that? Many people do.

It's okay for strong, survivor types to take medication too, you know.

Shame on Me

In 1977, Billy Joel released "Only the Good Die Young." Because I'm forever trying to lay blame, I want to hold him partially responsible for the horrible mistakes I made trying to gain the approval of boys and men after my dad left. I know it's really not Billy Joel's fault. He was only voicing one of many cultural myths we Americans tend to treat as fact.

Many years ago, as I drove down the road in my Chevy Malibu, I cranked up the radio and sang along. I was returning home from a visit with my father — a visit during which my father blamed my mother for their divorce. He told me, "In all the years we were married, your mother never made love to me. I always had to make love to her."

Besides feeling the shame of being a sought-after woman who wanted to avoid sex (at the tender age of seventeen), I also felt shame because I knew I was like my mother. How could I not have been like her? I was her daughter, and a woman. Similarities existed. I also got the creeps, because Dad had implied his new-found love was more sexually assertive than my mother had ever been. Well, I didn't need to know *that*. The seed had been planted for a still-lingering fear (yep, after all these years, I still have it) that my sexual behavior, or lack thereof, would someday cause *my* husband to leave *me*.

In his song, Billy urges Virginia not to wait, and so it was for me.

When I was sixteen, I dated a boy who insisted we go all the way. I refused. He moved on, like my father moved on from my mother. This confirmed my deepest fears.

Billy's song suggests girls should not wait to become sexually active.

I knew my boyfriend had had sex with other girls, even with my best friend. (Wasn't high school weird?) I was scared and, let's face it, full to the brim with self-loathing — after all, my dad had left me. And Dad had called me fat once. I could never let a boy see me naked. And besides, what was I expected to *do*? I felt so awkward.

Perhaps Billy's right — that it all comes down to fate.

By the time I left for college, I had promised another boy, who was a friend and with whom I had flirted for years, that I would have sex with him the next time I saw him. I was going away to college, and I naively didn't expect to ever see him again. Besides, the promise of sex in the future made him stop asking for sex that summer before college. Looking back, I must say that all the asking got really stressful. My breasts and other parts were in big demand. And boys sure do know how to demand, manipulate, and shame girls into sex.

So if it's gonna happen sooner or later, he may as well be the one.

Yeah, my friend was the one. When I came home for Christmas that first year of college, so did he. And he demanded. He begged. He told me I shouldn't break my promise.

And as for Billy's threat of the good dying young... well...

This is one of many, many lies I believed in my youth. Well, I don't know if I believed it. I just believed I should follow the cultural rules. Having been raised to be honest and keep my word, I think I actually felt I *should* give the boy what I had promised — my virginity. Besides, at this point I felt pressured and tired of being afraid of sex.

Merry Christmas. I drank a pitcher of beer, took a Quaalude, and made myself an honest woman. I even fixed him eggs for breakfast, not knowing what the protocol should be. Later, I couldn't get the blood stain off my mattress. It taunted me every wash day for years.

After I lost my virginity and went back to college, I was angry. I felt ashamed of what I had done. I realized on a very deep level that I had been an object of conquest for the boy, not a friend. By this time, my alcoholism was full blown, and I put myself in risky situation after risky situation. I began to act out my anger and self-loathing by inflicting sexual experiences on myself. I remember thinking, *Alright, you want to have sex with me? Here, have me. You only want one thing, so here it is.* As willing as I was to give men what they wanted, inside I was as cold as Mt. Everest. Numb.

These self-destructive acts seem grotesque to me now. I feel sad for the young woman who made those choices. It is only by the grace of God that I was able to leave her behind. But I didn't leave the shame behind. I have kept it with me all these years. First, the shame from my family, then the shame of my bad behavior, and finally the shame that I could not overcome my shame. Pretty hopeless, huh?

It's a good thing I have an equal part of me who wants to live with self-love and respect. She is the part of me who got sober and turned away from the *vida loca.* She is the one who fell in love with and married one of the least judgmental men a woman could find. These wonderful things in my life didn't completely erase my shame, but they certainly kept it from totally consuming me.

I have to forgive myself daily for the self-destructive mistakes I've made over the years. It is from that place of forgiveness that I have made my decision to have WLS. Maybe I am at a point in my life where I can finally and permanently let my little light shine. When I got sober, the light came on, but it was only forty watts or so. I tried to power it up with limited success (sixty watts, maybe), but I still felt dark and undeserving at the core. I continued to turn to food for nurturing and comfort, but now I know food is not my solution. It has long since stopped being a carefree comfort. It is killing me.

With almost every bite I take, I know my bulb is dimming. I have become so heavy, I have to pause and prepare emotionally and physically every time I get out of the car. Or out of a chair. Or off the toilet, for that matter. Sorry to be so graphic, but this is my life.

I have come to a deeper understanding of the shame and self-destructiveness I have had to deal with. I have tried to resolve my remaining issues over the years, but between my addiction to sugar, my depression, an abusive therapist (a long story not worth telling), and my willingness to set aside my needs so that I could take care of my needy family, I have gotten bogged down. Heavily bogged down — pun intended. And, of course, now I realize that a lot of my problems have been physical, not simply psychological.

Following the death of my mother, I also realize this life is not a dress rehearsal. I don't know how much time I have left on this earth. I know I don't want to spend that time feeling sick and sorry for myself. I want the light of the Creator to shine into my life and through my life. I have a strong urge to acknowledge the value of my life, my light and to use it for a greater good. (Okay, I also want to be able to sit at a table and lean in to play a game with Barrett without feeling pain in my stomach and throat because of the fat pressing up and pushing my stomach into my chest.) I'm hoping the surgery will get me up to a hundred watts or more! We'll see.

You'd think the stories of the physical pain my fat causes would be too shameful for me to tell. After all, most people think weight problems are caused by weak will and psychological problems. Most think it's my own fault if my weight causes me so much physical suffering. I have been shamed into that belief, and it has been a hard belief to let go of. I don't know if our culture ever will.

Some of the savvy doctors I have seen have said things similar to what my high-priced endocrinologist (who didn't accept insurance) told me years ago, and I just *couldn't* believe him.

He said, "You have a condition called insulin resistance. It makes it easier for you to gain weight and harder for you to lose weight. You didn't cause this condition."

Those words planted a seed, but other forces prevented me from letting them grow. I had almost completely succumbed to *the forces of shame.*

I've always felt guilty for my successes in life. I happened to develop earlier than Sarah — both physically and academically. While she has gone on to achieve amazing things in her career and maintained a naturally slender figure to boot, Sarah suffered in her youth as I came home with blue ribbons and A pluses. I'm not sure how my parents handled all that, but I know Sarah felt stupid and weak. She tried to feel better about herself by putting me down. She joined my parents in criticizing me — Scapegoat Katie, the big black sheep. And I responded by working hard to keep that grim title for many years.

When I look back at how dysfunctional my parents were, I really don't blame Sarah for her harshness. I think my father told her she was the pretty one and I was the smart one. Helpful, eh? It was an insult to both of us. The joke was on Dad, though. Sarah is a beauty, and she's smart. Sharp. Savvy. Successful. And I am smart and quite beautiful in my own way, if I do say so myself.

I wanted Sarah to love me when we were kids, but she considered me the enemy. It has taken years for us to get past that. But I still feel guilty when I am successful. And she still says and does things that hurt me. And I still embarrass her at times. Maybe we've moved from dysfunctional sisters to garden-variety sisters. That's my goal.

I don't only feel guilty when I do well in relation to Sarah. I also feel embarrassed when I get too far ahead in a board game. Once, when my husband and I were playing Pictionary with friends, we were getting way ahead, so I leaned over to Mike and actually whispered, "We're too far ahead! I don't want people to get mad at us." My husband, the former competitive swimmer, looked at me as if I were an alien.

When I first started dating my husband, we went to a big picnic and joined a group playing croquet on the front lawn. When it was Mike's turn, he hit his ball close to someone else's and for his next stroke sent their ball careening across that yard and the neighbor's. I was furious and embarrassed for him and for myself. I almost broke up with him over that game. I didn't understand how anyone could be so comfortable with playing so ruthlessly. Mike pointed out he was playing the game by the rules. I fumed.

I felt so different from Mike and maybe even a bit scared by his confidence. I began to question whether I could continue to date him, but I was seriously attracted to him. I had already fallen in love actually. So, I made him join a couple's support group with me (so that he could work on *his problems*). We spent the next five years meeting every Saturday night with that group, and we both changed a lot. The couple's group saw us through our engagement, our marriage, and the birth of our son. I have no doubt we would not be together today if it hadn't been for that group.

And despite our major differences, Mike and I have learned to treat each other with respect. It wasn't that we were perfect; we just were willing to admit our weaknesses and try to do better. We learned to apologize and forgive each other as often as necessary. That has been a great recipe for us.

Speaking of Recipes

I will miss pigging out with Mike. We sure have enjoyed eating together over the years. Our first restaurant was one we called the "Hey, Lady" restaurant, because the owner always greeted me with, "Hey, Lady!"

Mike and I held hands across the pink tablecloth and talked about our dreams there, and then we polished off two or three orders of Chinese delights. Then we found the Peking Gourmet Inn, which was President George H. W. Bush's favorite restaurant at the time — or so I've heard. We never saw him there, but the food was great! We also loved Generous George's Positive Pizza Place. Good memories.

Will I have no more happy, food-related memories? I just don't know. I worry that if I go to restaurants too often or continue to make eating a hobby I share with my husband, I will *eat through the surgery. Eating through the surgery* means overeating after you've had the surgery so that you gain your weight back, or worse, you damage your stomach and staple line. Very scary.

Now that we've been married more than fifteen years and have an eleven-year-old son, we don't pig out as much as we used to. Mike seems more than willing to change our relationship with food to help me lose weight and feel better. He is supportive of the WLS but afraid of complications, afraid of losing me. I admit I'm scared too. Terrified, actually. The surgeons are quite optimistic, however, so I became willing to consider it. Plus, I am so very tired of feeling awful.

I had never seriously considered WLS until a surgeon who was going to remove my gall bladder suggested gastric bypass in addition to the gall bladder removal.

The surgeon was warm and friendly, which surprised me, considering my track record for finding compassionate doctors. During the examination part of my consultation, the surgeon didn't mention WLS. He confirmed that I was a good candidate for the gall bladder surgery and said he'd be happy to do it. Being terrified of surgery, I asked the doctor if I would have a better chance at a good outcome if I lost weight before the surgery.

As I lay down on the examination table feeling huge and ashamed, the surgeon pressed around on my stomach and said in a most grandfatherly tone (as he sat me up and patted my hand), "I have operated on people a lot heavier than you, sweetheart.

Don't worry. I'll take good care of you and you'll do just fine. But, since you bring up your weight, let's go talk in my office."

I can't really remember if he called me sweetheart, but it *felt* like he did. Grandfathers can be so comforting — at least the ones in my imagination.

Confused, I followed the surgeon to his office. He said something like, "You know, a person your size usually has a very difficult time losing weight and keeping it off. Your body is working against you at this point. You are young, and considering your size, you are relatively healthy now. You should consider gastric bypass surgery. They could take out your gall bladder at the same time, so you would only have to have one operation."

I sat speechless.

The surgeon continued, "I don't do the surgery myself. You should go talk to a surgeon I know who does weight loss surgery. He's been doing it for many years and he does a good job."

"I never considered gastric bypass," I mumbled. *Was I that bad?* (Only my own denial would have allowed me to ask myself *that* question.)

"Some people worry about this surgery. But if you try to lose weight and fail again, you'll just be older, probably even more overweight, and sicker the next time you consider the surgery."

"Isn't it dangerous?" I squeaked.

"There will never be a better time in your life to have gastric bypass. Go to an experienced surgeon who has been doing the procedure for years, and you'll be fine."

I had never considered WLS before that day. I left the surgeon's office stunned.

It's All My Fault

I have always believed that my weight gain is all my fault and that I should be able to work through my issues and lose it. Since I believed that I had caused it, I also believed I had to correct whatever psychological dysfunction I had, or I would never lose weight and keep it off. That is what led me to admit myself to a psychiatric hospital for binge eating disorder treatment in the year 2000. Welcome to the new millennium.

The treatment was useless for the most part — except that I got a good lesson in compassion. I learned a lot about bulimia and anorexia, and the staff primarily focused on the bulimics and anorexics. The people suffering from those diseases were heartbreaking. They were wounded and hurting and close to death. Maybe I was too, but my death wasn't quite as imminent, and the staff acted accordingly. Despite my thoughts of suicide, I wasn't as critical as the others. The staff's lack of attention was disappointing and confirmed my sense of worthlessness. My insurance was paying the same $40,000 a month the other patients' insurances were paying.

I participated in the program with as much earnestness as I could muster, but ultimately that hospitalization was not effective for me. I felt like I was as annoying to the staff as I had been to my family years ago. I needed more than they could give me. Always more. "Katie, the game is over."

The one thing I did learn at the treatment center was that I needed to go on — and stay on — antidepressants, and they have made a world of difference in my life. Oh yeah, I learned one other thing — trying to lose weight was hopeless.

I had been fooled by a myth about obesity that tricks many people — *my mental weaknesses and sinful, gluttonous behavior was the sole cause of my weight problem, and I was a hopeless case.*

I know now that this is simply not true. In large part, my weight problem is caused by genetics, years of yo-yo dieting, and my diabetes (insulin resistance). There is a psychological component, but so many other factors contribute to obesity. It's complicated, simply complicated.

There is a debate raging about food and addiction. Some people, including me, feel they are addicted to food, especially sugar and refined carbs. A friend, who happens to be a scientist, swears sugar is not addictive — at least not in the same sense as alcohol and drugs. I won't be surprised if she's proven wrong, but in the meantime, psychological addiction has to be factored into a recovery from obesity.

When I look back at my years of dieting, twelve-step programs, and hospitalizations, I realize my mental health has been affected. I turned a lack of nurturing and my love of food into an eating disorder. How did this happen? I've thought a lot about that.

For a long time, I thought I just had an addictive personality. I thought I was self-destructive and a weak-willed, worthless person who couldn't get control of herself. Now I believe that the culture of shame that surrounds fat in America actually contributes to the development of eating disorders. Most of America's fat is caused by an overabundance of sugary, refined foods; ignorance about nutrition; television with too many yummy commercials; and the constant shaming of our bodies — we're just never perfect enough.

Dieting is a Catch-22. It makes us skinny for awhile, but then we get hungry on a very deep level. We feel deprived, as those around us in commercials and in real life encourage us to eat sweets and junk food. Slipping off the dieting bandwagon causes shame, self-loathing, and more weight gain. Not just because of our eating disorders, though. We have been fighting the subtle commands of our body as well. Again, we know that *95–98 percent of the time, dieting ultimately causes weight gain.* Numerous studies have proven that dieting causes weight gain in the long run. That certainly happened to me.

I also know that food has comforted me for many years, and the habit of seeking comfort in food started when I was really young — and really needy.

I heard a savvy bariatric surgeon on a radio show coach a slightly overweight woman to accept herself as she was instead of dieting. I was shocked. Would I have stayed reasonably small (not thin, but not morbidly obese either) if a doctor had told me to stop dieting and maintain my weight at 180 pounds? I could have done pretty well at that weight, as long as I stayed active and ate enough nutritious foods.

But no. I thought weighing 180 pounds was shameful. Sarah and Mom certainly thought so. I just think of all the fun I could have had over the years at a weight that still allowed me to move comfortably and shop in regular stores — a weight that didn't hinder my desire to be active and productive.

But that's water under the bridge now. I am grateful that at least I have the option of surgery. I just need to make sure I don't let my eating disorder affect my success. I am going to work like hell. And with the surgery, much less effort will be required to avoid overeating. Or so I'm told.

When Mike and I walked into the WLS surgeon's office, the first thing I noticed were the large chairs in the waiting room. What a concept: chairs that I didn't have to squeeze my butt into. As I sat there like Edith Ann (I have short legs that didn't touch the ground when I sat back in the chair), I felt a million butterflies darting around my stomach. They took flight each time the nurse came out and called a name. Mike sat beside me, taking it all in. He was nervous too.

We only spent about ten minutes with the WLS surgeon, but he answered all our questions. Mike looked as white as a ghost during the whole visit, and I know he was freaked out. I was too. Even though people have surgery every day, I was scared. Today, when I visited an online message board for people having WLS, there was a memorial message for a WLS patient who had died of a blood clot. That freaks me out!

Mike and I were talking as if I had decided to go ahead with the surgery. After meeting with the WLS surgeon, I told Mike I was keeping an open mind and would not rush a decision. The next day I started talking about the logistics of having surgery and Mike just carried on the conversation with me unquestioningly. I really don't have any choice if I want to lead a better life. I just wish people didn't ever die from this treatment.

It isn't normally my nature to insist on doing something that Mike disapproves of, but I realize I can't base my decision on his permission alone. I have to make this decision for myself and accept the consequences.

Some days I think about how much I'll miss eating. This morning, I woke up thinking about cake. I will miss cake quite a bit. Over the weekend, we ate out a lot. I realized we spent a lot of the weekend planning what to eat and eating. What will I do with all that free time once I have the surgery? I won't be able to think about food all the time unless I want to totally torture myself.

It's time to admit it to myself — I've made the decision to have the surgery. Now I'm feeling an intense mixture of excitement and dread.

The Attitude Diet

I have been a negative, critical thinker for a long, long time. I
come by it honestly. My mother was the same way. Nothing is ever
as satisfying as it could be and that feeling of what could have
been is almost always my dominant thought. I wonder if the negative thinking is just a habit to be broken. I have always struggled
with depression. Has that brought on the negative thinking? I actually
have existential depression. Depression about the big questions and
absurdities in life that are unresolvable. (I told you I'm complicated.) I
really need to work on what I allow myself to think about. I worry, will I
be able to control my attitude or will my attitude control me?

I will have to go on an attitude diet. One day at a time, one
minute at a time, I will have to change my thinking, hoping that will

change my attitude. I will treat it like a diet, hoping that I won't regain my negative thinking, plus a little more, once I lose it.

This morning Barrett asked me, "Mom? What's *ironic?*" What a loaded question. I know he meant what does ironic *mean.* I couldn't tell him the definition. I could use the word in a sentence, but I had to look up the actual meaning.

Irony is a close companion of complicated people like me. It's ironic that I'm a clinical social worker (counselor) who struggles with depression and neurosis. It's ironic that I have immense willpower but cannot maintain weight loss. It's ironic that I have done so many diets and therapies, yet I'm still fat.

America's relationship with food has ironies as well. It's ironic that the media and government are putting out daily TV news and news magazine stories about how obese Americans are getting, and yet there are food commercials sprinkled throughout the broadcasts. It's ironic that gastric bypass has been a viable treatment for morbidly obese patients for years and that I have been directly asking my doctors for help for years, and yet not one of my doctors ever suggested WLS to me until the gallbladder surgeon. It's ironic that I suffered numerous miscarriages in my thirties and could have had gastric bypass (which increases the likelihood of successful pregnancies) but was not referred for the surgery by any of my many doctors.

Assuming the WLS is a success and I wait the two years I'm supposed to wait before trying for another child, I would be forty-seven before I would even be able to deliver a baby. And that's too old for me, especially in the sense that Barrett would be in high school by then, and it would be hard to go back to changing diapers.

My son would have loved to have had a sibling close to his age and I would have loved that too.

In my thirties, I was almost as obese as I am now but healthier. I had already lost and regained a hundred pounds twice. I had a body mass index of more than forty (one of the criteria for surgery). I can only imagine how my life would have been different if I had had WLS then.

The depth of my pain resulting from the loss of the opportunity to have more children is almost unbearable right now. I ache for the babies I lost through miscarriage and the ones I could have had. It's ironic that in a few months my body will begin to heal and become fertile and healthy, but it will be too late to have more children.

I didn't know what to expect at the appointment with my surgeon's nurse following my decision to have WLS. My butterflies returned as I entered the office. A group of large people sat in the oversize chairs. They were chatting. Two had had their surgeries the week before and sought to reassure the rest of us. I kept my mouth shut at first — too shy to add anything, too embarrassed to be there.

I was called in after a twenty-minute wait. I was given a pre-op checklist, and the physician's assistant went over the lab work I would need to have done. That was it. Five minutes! From the surgeon's perspective, this was no big deal. I, on the other hand, was quietly freaking out.

The insurance issues related to WLS are frustrating. Despite the fact that I have coverage for surgery, the insurance company reserves the right to find a loophole and not pay for the procedure. Plus, they may not cover the surgical assistant or perhaps some of the lab work. It's crazy. What I don't understand is why we as a nation put up with the way the insurance companies treat us. When I call, it almost seems like they are hard to reach on purpose. I almost never get all my questions answered. I almost always have to get transferred and listen to endless recordings and instructions, only to be disconnected in the end. I spent an hour on the phone this morning in the maze of my insurance company's menus and had to quit after getting only one of three questions answered. Why *do* we put up with this?

Will I be able to eat baked potatoes after the surgery? I know I won't be able to eat them right away, but what about six months down the road? I guess the quantity will have to be much, much smaller, like a quarter of a baked potato, *after* I eat my protein. I will miss eating a big, old baked potato. All that butter, salt, and pepper — oh, and sour cream. Yesterday, I actually teared up thinking about how I will never again eat a whole baked potato once I have the surgery. To me, potatoes are *da bomb*.

Food has such a deep-seated power to comfort me. How will I comfort myself without baked potatoes? I know it sounds a bit absurd, but that *is* one of the million-dollar questions. My overeating is primarily for comfort. Yes, sometimes it's celebratory, and sometimes it's to stuff feelings, but mostly it's to quell a general discomfort with my life. It fills a vague emotional void I seem to have. Usually, I eat because I need to be nurtured or I feel a touch of hopelessness or occasionally because I'm feeling some type of loss. The thought of having to nurture and fill myself with something other than food is beyond depressing.

The truth is, for a while after the surgery, I'll have this cold, sad lump in my throat, not a warm potato. I'll have to find other ways to satisfy myself, but let's face it — a bubble bath is not a bowl of ice cream topped with Spanish peanuts. Journaling is not that extra dollop of sour cream on my chili. Taking a nature walk does not envelop me in a gentle calm the way my mom's chicken a lá king on biscuits does. And okay, I admit it, sex is not a piece of chocolate cake.

I've been reading WLS message boards online, and someone asked if sex was better after the surgery. The answer was a resounding YES. Apparently, size does matter. My body size. Of course, when I'm smaller, I'll be more comfortable. That's what the people who've had the surgery have experienced. They have more energy and feel better about themselves (even *with* the sagging skin that develops with rapid weight loss), and several people said they find sex much more pleasurable.

Frankly, nothing physical that I do feels very good at this point. I am so uncomfortable from my weight almost everything feels too painful. My reflux is so bad, for example, I can't put any pressure on my stomach, because the food I've eaten pushes up into my esophagus. Kinda dampens the sex drive.

I also feel a lot of shame, despite a very loving husband who understands and accepts the complexity of my health situation. Much to my constant amazement, he continues to be attracted to me. And after surgery when I feel better, I'm sure we'll have a much better time in bed.

I'm not just hoping for better sex though. I also want better intimacy. I have always wanted more attention from my husband in general. But I also know that when he is available, I get very nervous under his scrutiny. It's like I want him, but the moment I have him, I get nervous and turn away. On a therapist's couch when I was in my twenties, I learned about how the loss of my father through divorce was such a deep betrayal that I have had trouble allowing anyone to get too close. Also, my self-loathing runs deep. But I don't want to do the dance of shame anymore, even though I am terrified to change my steps. I need to give it a try despite my fears. I'm sure my husband will be willing to learn a new dance.

Even in the first few years of our relationship, I gained almost a hundred pounds, struggled through a major weight loss, and regained the weight, plus a little. Actually, I did that twice! After the second of those weight losses and the beginning of the subsequent weight gain, Mike and I sat down for a serious talk at my request. As we held hands across the table at "Hey, Lady," I teared up as I told Mike how sorry I was that he married a woman with an eating disorder and weight problem. (I had not been fat when he met me.) We'd been married a few years, and I was doing the yo-yo thing again. I was discouraged and confused. I didn't want to gain the weight back. I was heartbroken and felt helpless.

"I can't seem to control my weight. I know it must be hard to have a fat wife. I'm so sorry." I was crying as I said this.

Mike reached across the table to hold my hands, "I've seen you struggle. I've witnessed your amazing willpower. I have known for a long time that something is wrong with you that is not completely in your control."

I cried as we looked into each other's eyes intensely. (So intensely I felt exposed and embarrassed.)

He continued, "I see the magazines and TV shows with thin women. I admit those women are attractive. But they are a fantasy. A fantasy. And I'm very much in love with my reality."

Oh, my. Now that kind of unconditional love is definitely better than a baked potato.

10

Hopes and Doubts and Fears, Oh My!

Maybe it's my ADHD-esque tendencies. Maybe it's my deep longing to be taken care of (the way my parents rarely took care of me). Maybe it is self-loathing buried in layers of fat. Maybe it's pure laziness. I don't know. But I've never consistently taken good care of myself or set enough limits with myself. It's embarrassing to admit, but something fundamental in my character is sabotaging my life.

Last year, I decided it would be nice to teach Barrett some lessons about character. I checked out a children's book at the library about self-discipline along with a lot of other interesting books.

Each night I would lay out the books in front of Barrett so that he could choose one for me to read to him. Each night he gleefully picked any book but the one on self-discipline. After I'd read all the other books to him, I finally insisted on reading the self-discipline book to him. He was mad. Yet, like a good little bibliophile, he snuggled up next to me for storytime — but kept his head turned away from me. Humph!

I began reading the book in my best dramatic story-telling voice, but before I'd gotten to page two, Barrett's shoulders started to shake. Then I heard a squeak and then an all-out sob.

"What's wrong?" I gently grasped his shoulders and turned him to face me.

"I," he sniffed, "hate," sniff, sniff, "self," sniff, sniff, "discipline," and then he just collapsed and sobbed for a good minute.

The funny thing was, I knew exactly how he felt. *I hate it too*, I thought. But, of course, I didn't tell him that. I went straight to feeling guilty and ashamed. Barrett is so much like me, it hurts sometimes. We never did finish the book.

My physically inactive life has rubbed off on Barrett. As he heads toward puberty, he has adopted a sedentary lifestyle that I have not worked against — I really have no excuse. When he was younger, he was somewhat hyperactive, which kept him slimmer. And now, as I have gotten fatter, the fact that he's slowed down in the hyperactive department has been a relief, but it has not been a great benefit to him.

During the year my mom was living with us, my sweet son slowly increased his TV viewing during the day, knowing I wasn't available to him the way I used to be. And because I had so little time for myself, I increased my TV viewing at night to escape the stress I was feeling and to zone out for awhile. I ate chocolate ice cream with Jay Leno or Ted Koppel every night before bed.

Barrett increased his intake of carbohydrates and his mindless eating. (Mind you, he's not fat, but he carries a lot more fat on his body than he used to.) Maybe it's normal for a kid to gain some weight as he approaches puberty. I have no idea what normal is. What if he is addicted to carbs? What if we're too sedentary? Okay, I know those things are true, whether puberty is playing a role or not.

I just *hate* self-discipline.

I seem to be in a cycle of feeling hope, then doubt, then fear. It's clear that there can be complications with surgery, and recovery is not always a piece of cake (sorry, pun intended).

I worry that I will go through yet another gut-wrenching (okay, yes, another pun intended) weight loss process, only to regain the weight. The truth is — the surgery is not a cure. People sometimes gain their weight back. Not everyone, but enough people do that it scares me. I am too old to go through another failure. (Although didn't someone say if you haven't failed, you haven't really lived?)

I told someone awhile back that I didn't want to diet again because I didn't think I had it in me, from an emotional standpoint, to go through another weight gain. It's just so devastating. The amount of willpower it takes to do the kind of dieting I did is staggering. And that makes the weight regain all the more painful. When I lost weight in a twelve-step program, I went for an entire year without sugar and white flour. I still can't believe I returned to my old ways and began to overeat again. I don't know why I didn't embrace my lifestyle change permanently.

I have to figure out why I failed, or I fear I am doomed to repeat my mistakes. And the surgery sounds just unpleasant enough that I don't want to go through it if I'm not 100 percent sure I'm going to succeed afterward. Frankly, why put my life at risk for nothing?

I can't even remember what year I abstained from sugar and white flour. Hmmmmm. Oh yeah, it was right after I got married. I had gone on a starvation diet before the wedding, then I got fat again. Then I started working the twelve steps. I went to daily meetings, got a sponsor, and followed directions — just like they tell you to. So why did I ultimately fail?

I was also in "family-of-origin therapy" (you know, the therapy through which we come to terms with the dysfunctional family of our childhood) right before I married. I went to my therapy group once a week and discussed how growing up in a dysfunctional family caused me to have such self-loathing and self-destructive behavior. I learned about shame and shared my pain.

I had lost about a hundred pounds and had just gotten married when the group ended. One of our members had died of AIDS, I had started a new life, and the therapist thought our group should be "done." I can remember her walking me to the door while telling me to go live my life, go enjoy what I'd worked so hard for. I told her I felt like something was still wrong with me. Something deep inside still didn't feel right.

"Off you go," she said. "You are a beautiful, strong woman. Go live your life."

I was already gaining the weight back as that therapist pushed me out the door. I wish I had listened to my inner voice and gotten more help. I knew I wasn't cured.

In the twelve-step meetings, I felt ashamed. When you are losing weight, everyone calls you a winner during the meetings. They say things like, "Stick with the winners." Even though it was supposed to be a spiritual program, weight loss was equated with success. There were people there who understood my struggles and commiserated with me. They were regaining too. But the ones who were losing or maintaining a loss were considered the "goddesses." They were the ones people went to for help. When they talked, people felt inspired.

Some of them were absolute successes — that 2–5 percent who actually kept the weight off. The rest of them were people who were on the falling side of the yo-yo cycle. One woman in particular really upset me, because I knew there was no cure, but she was acting righteous and cured.

"I am so frustrated," I shared, as we sat around a little table in a church classroom in little plastic chairs. (Talk about a sore butt.) "I want to be abstinent, but I just can't seem to stop overeating."

Several other people at the meeting sympathized with me and offered what little inspiration they could. Looking back, I realize that probably no one at that particular meeting had had long-term weight loss. But one proud woman, who had recently lost a hundred pounds, approached me after the meeting and hugged me.

She said, "Oh, I have been where you are." Hug, hug. Pity, pity. She didn't know I had already lost a hundred pounds before my regain.

Here's what I thought and will forever wish I had said to that woman when she told me she had been where I was. I thought, *How do you know I'm not where you're going?* What made her think she was cured? The pink cloud of weight loss can bring on a lot of magical thinking. A lot.

The million-dollar question is whether WLS will set me back on the same pink cloud — the one I have always fallen off of.

Actually, there is another million-dollar question. How have I managed to stay away from alcohol and cigarettes all these years? I did both for more than ten years, and then I quit both. What was different?

The Art of Setting Boundaries

I have to learn to take time for me. Why is this so tricky? I mean, that is the key, isn't it? With my mother dying and my own health so poor, I hadn't done a lot of homeschooling with Barrett during the year, which is why I put him in a school that works with special needs kids (he struggles with dyslexia and dysgraphia). I didn't want the year to be a total loss, and I wanted to spend some time thinking about what *I* needed to lose. It is such a profound relief to have long periods of time to myself. Hey! I started writing again!

I have made all the phone calls I need to make, I have puttered around the house a bit, and I have relaxed my way through a spring head cold that I would have had to trudge through in other years. I haven't seen my friends a lot. Haven't talked to them on the phone much. Looking back, I realize I have been using my friendships to keep busy instead of busying myself with taking care of my problems. The irony is, I'm having a great time. I don't feel lonely. Now seeing my friends is a treat instead of an escape. This extrovert is reformed!

I don't need my husband and son with me every minute either. It's kind of funny. Mike spent lots of time traveling back and forth to North Carolina to be with his mother during her final months. Then, after she died, Mike immediately signed up for twelve hours worth of college courses to prepare him for a second master's degree. I complained a lot during the school part of his absence from home, because I thought he should devote himself to Barrett and me once his mom died. Okay, the funny part is, now that his classes are over and he's home all the time, he's driving me crazy.

It's hard to get used to having to pay attention to Mike and *his* needs in addition to my needs and Barrett's. I'll get used to him again, but having him underfoot makes me aware of how much I need to work on setting boundaries.

It's not that I don't want to exercise. I just don't want to put myself in a position in which some misunderstanding soul thinks she's trying to help me but is not. I am not motivated by shame, by being weighed by skinny people, by listing what I have eaten so others can evaluate my choices. My decision to go ahead with WLS and my willingness to follow the rules that go with the surgery is my decision to change. If other people can't see my pure heart and they want to police me, that's not my problem.

I want to exercise. I just don't want anyone at the gym to say, "Come in a few minutes early so we can weigh and measure you" — especially after I've told that person those tactics don't work for me. I am uncomfortable with being weighed and measured; it makes me feel ashamed, and shame is not a motivator for me — in fact, it repels me. The gym worker who wanted to weigh me said she wanted to help me and she would feel badly if I didn't come in. And I thought, *Excuse me! It's not my job to make you feel good.*

I don't care if she felt like she failed with me. She was pressuring me and attempting to control me so that she could feel good about helping someone. If she were being honest, she would have told me she didn't believe I had made the decision to change and would only believe it if she could see it and manage it. (Of course, I might have had to slap her if she'd actually said that.)

Why are we taught to be nice instead of taught to take care of ourselves? How many of us have put ourselves in unsafe situations because we were more worried about hurting someone's feelings than about our own well being?

Once you start paying attention, you may find your boundaries are being violated on a regular basis. Awhile back, I told a friend I was trying to lose weight. The next time we got our children together for a playdate at the park, she brought cookies "for the kids," although she ate some too. That was a violation of my boundaries, and I should have taken Barrett and left. Why associate with people who don't respect me? After surgery, I want to be stronger and reject those kinds of "friends."

When I quit drinking, I took my mother to a wedding with me for moral support. I was still new to sobriety and felt uncomfortable with the drinking that I knew would go on at the reception.

Ironically, that is one of the few times in my life that my mother got tipsy in public. I was so enraged and hurt.

After I have WLS, I'll continue to experience boundary violations. There are great books about how to improve one's boundary setting and I plan to re-read them. I believe being willing to set boundaries will be directly related to my success with WLS.

I heard on the news yesterday that the World Health Organization announced that no more than 10 percent of a diet should consist of sugar or other sweeteners. Of course, the sugar industry doesn't agree. That is no surprise to me. I think people are addicted to sugar and I think the food industry understands and uses that to its advantage.

The reason the food industry doesn't take a lot of heat for adding sugar to so many products is that sugar is sweet. Criticizing sugar is like kicking puppies.

Oh sweet sugar, you make candy and other treats! (You used to be added to cigarette tobacco.) I think we trivialize the danger of sugar because we associate it with motherhood and apple pie. Mmmmmmmm. Apple pie has lots of sugar!

It's insidious. My nephew's friends don't think the latest video game is cool. They think it's *SWEET*. When someone is nice, we don't call them bitter — we call them *sweet*. We have images of sugar plums in our heads; we call our loved ones sugar-pie-honey-bunch, sugar foot (that's what my mom called me), or sweetheart. Some of us even have sweetie pies.

Fat has robbed me of a lot of things — one of the main things is the ability to achieve my dreams. I don't know why this big body has been useful to me. Maybe I have been afraid to live my dreams and it gives me the excuse I need. The thing is, if I don't get busy, I'm going to die without living my dreams. I realize real life constrains us sometimes. No matter what was going on in my life when my mom came to our house to die, I had to set aside some of my dreams for awhile.

There are many times, however, when it would be just as easy to live my dreams as it would be to spend time doing things I *have* to do. Hear me out.

How many of us say, "I have to..." all the time?

"Oh honey, I'd love to do that, but I *have to* drop off this casserole at Mariane's house."

"I'd love to, but I *have to* finish this cross-stitch for my new niece."

"I wish I could have done that, but Rachel had a birthday party, and I *had to* spend two hours running from store to store looking for some doll all her friends have."

Do we really *have to*? One of my friends says it all the time. Granted, she is a giving person who contributes to her community in numerous ways. She is active in her church and nurturing to her friends. But every time I talk to her, I ask, "How are you?" She usually says, "I'm tired." I have said the same many times in my life.

I'm not saying my friend shouldn't contribute her good works to the world. I'm just saying, how much is it costing her? And, is there something she can contribute that is less expensive in time, money, and effort that would be just as valuable?

Could it be that taking care of ourselves contributes to the world? Isn't it a relief not to have to take care of someone because they choose to take care of themselves? That's a contribution.

My mother, God bless her, came to live with us at a time in her life when she had become dependent on alcohol for comfort. She smoked too and moved in thinking it'd be okay to continue with her self-destructive lifestyle in my home. At first, we tried to accommodate her, but then I started finding her in bed at night smoking, and the next morning she would deny she had been doing that. Blackouts. We had to come together as a family and confront my mother so that she would stop smoking in the house and cut down on her drinking.

What would life have been like in her final year if she had been taking care of herself? If she had recognized and owned her problems and taken care of herself instead of behaving like a victim? Unfortunately, she passed that lovely *victim* trait on to me. I have to work so hard to *not* be a victim. It's such a familiar place to go. I've fought it long and hard. Mostly because I don't want to teach Barrett to be a victim and give up the way my mother did and the way I have on occasion. Wow, it hurts to say *that*.

Even my mom's cancer would probably have been curable if she had been willing to take care of herself instead of be victimized. Her breast cancer was diagnosed long after it could have been, and it probably had been detected by my mom. I don't know if she was depressed, or felt unworthy, or was lonely. I don't know.

She did things that pushed us away. Maybe she didn't feel worthy.

That is a legacy I don't want. Choosing WLS is choosing to finally step up and take care of myself instead of taking care of the world. Many of us just have our priorities wrong.

When an airplane loses altitude and there is a sudden loss of cabin pressure, we are told to put on our own oxygen mask first and then help the person next to us. Is your own oxygen mask firmly in place? Is mine? No! And that is what has to change.

In my dreams, I have all the oxygen I need, and I am soaring. In reality, the things I want to do are quite attainable. The feeling-proud dreams, the feeling-accomplished dreams — those are within reach. Even the getting-rich dreams, if that's what I really want.

Some people reading this will think, *Yeah, sure, you can "fulfill your dreams," but I have to take care of my disabled child (or some other genuinely challenging situation).* I don't believe, however, that any situation is hopeless.

We must ask ourselves, "What is available to me that I have not asked for or accepted?"

"What would be available if I made minor adjustments in my life to make room for what I need?"

"What major changes could I make that would make my life easier?"

"Are the roadblocks in my life created in my mind by telling myself 'I *have* to' or 'I *should*'?"

"What are my goals?"

I read once that the vast majority of people who actually write down their specific goals achieve them. It's not rocket science. Goals are achievable. I'm going to write that down on a card and tape it to my mirror.

A Flurry of Feelings

Because I decided not to rush into an irreversible decision, and such a big one at that, I have given myself permission to take the slow road to WLS surgery. Being an impulsive person, waiting more than two months for surgery is stressful. I want it to be over with. At the same time, I don't want it to ever come. I still have so much fear about the surgery. I worry that I won't survive it. Or I will have complications. I worry I will suffer long after the surgery is over. Most people do just fine, I know. But enough people have complications that I am obsessing about it.

I wonder if I should write a letter to Barrett in case I don't survive the surgery. Now that's a gloomy thought.

I told my husband he has to forgive me if I die from the surgery. He said he'd have to get a lot of therapy. Sarah doesn't seem to have any qualms about the surgery. She wants me to be around for a long time, and she worries more about what the weight is doing to me.

Life is so precious to me. I wish I'd never gotten to this point in the first place.

I don't want to dwell on my anxious feelings too much. I also have hopeful feelings. I can't wait to feel good. I can't wait for the day when every step I take is not a burden. So much of everyday life is a chore to me; I can't wait for things to get easier. Like stopping at the grocery store for a couple of things. Or walking from the parking lot to my doctor's office. Or even getting up to answer the front door. Or showering. It's all hard now. As I've gotten bigger, my life has gotten smaller.

I wonder what I'll do with all my newfound energy once I recover from surgery. When I am feeling good, I'm a bit hyper. I am intense, and I don't know how to be that way as an adult in this world. I think it's always been hard for me to harness my energy, my restlessness. Now, of course, it's all mental, but when I'm thinner and healthier, it will be physical too. I think weight and food have helped me be more subdued, and I have to have a plan to deal with my energy when it comes back. I'm certainly going to have to find some new hobbies.

I think you can tell a lot about people by the songs they have connected with over their lifetime. My mother, for example, loved the song "Yesterday" by Roy Clark. You know, "Yesterday, when I was young…"

Mom never got over yesterday. She died with yesterday unresolved.

Now me, I have a whole list of songs I have been drawn to over the years. And they reflect my significant emotional stages. As a pre-teen, I listened to forty-fives. Sarah and I would take the bus downtown and buy records of our favorite songs. I had a recliner in my bedroom and I would lounge in it, sing loudly along with my songs, cry, and daydream about Davy Jones, Bobby Sherman, Donnie Osmond, and other *Tiger Beat* favorites.

I actually still have my collection of forty-fives. My real favorites were the sad, sappy songs like "Never My Love" and "Everything I Own," which made me cry hard every time I listened to them after my dad left.

By early high school, I wept to "Your Song" by Elton John and "Don't Take Your Love Away from Me" by Neil Sedaka. I was an emotional basket case.

My devastating losses began when my dad left, but they continued. My parents had belonged to a country club before Dad left, and after he left, he began taking his new love to the club, knowing full well Mom's community was there. This was very hard on my mom, of course, and she dealt with it by moving us across the country.

I remember sitting on the black and white Spanish-style couch in our living room looking at a map of the United States with Mom and Sarah. Mom was showing us where Seattle is (we were living on the East Coast at the time). We decided to drive across the country and start a new life where our cousins lived, near Lake Washington.

When all this decision-making was going on, I was trying to have the best year of school in my whole short life, but my family crisis was ruining it. I loved cheerleading. I liked the dance routines, the precision, the athletics, the competition, and the popularity.

Then I learned how shallow kids can be. My friends quickly grew sick of my sadness about my parents' breakup. What little confidence I had with boys vanished when my dad left. In my mind, I was unworthy and unlovable. And nothing seemed fun anymore. My parents seemed totally disengaged from my life, and I didn't know how to handle the mix of emotions swirling inside me.

Then we moved. I felt sad saying goodbye to all my friends, even though they did not offer a lot of comfort. At my going-away party, they were so busy socializing, as freshmen will do, that I did not get a whole lot of attention. One girl I hadn't even met before stands out in my memory. She had just moved back from overseas and offered the only words of compassion I got that evening.

"You'll be okay," she said. "It's hard to go, but you'll make lots of new friends and you will have fun again. I promise."

I felt warm inside. I felt understood. I also felt a new sadness, because I could not pursue a friendship with the one person who seemed to understand me.

In Seattle, I got a new lease on my young life. I really loved it there, but Mom and Sarah didn't. So, after eleven months, we returned to the East Coast, moving to a new neighborhood, which meant that we didn't return to our original high school.

This second move just about did me in. The good-bye was even more devastating than the one from my first move. As I stood on a beach in the Pacific Northwest at the cast party following the school play, my boyfriend and I held hands and faced into the wind, watching screeching girls and splashing guys laugh together in the gray ocean waves. I didn't want to go swimming. I hated my body and was ashamed to be seen in my swimsuit. (My intense shame has caused me to miss out on a lot of things.) I didn't feel like laughing with the kids anyway.

I was standing slightly in front of my boyfriend and down a little from the frolicking kids, so no one could see my tears. The wind swallowed my sobs. I knew that when I moved away, none of these kids would remember I had ever lived there. I imagined their happy lives would continue on, while I suffered more loss and hopelessness.

I think I stayed in Seattle a month or so longer than my mom and sister. I remember I stayed with my closest friends for a while before I headed east again. At Kristen's house, I slept on the floor and hung out in her room. I didn't see her parents much. But I remember sitting next to her stereo, crying (yet again), and listening to Elton John's "Your Song" while I heard Kristen arguing with her parents down the hall.

I remember Kristen yelling, "She has to stay with us, Mom. She doesn't have any place else to go!"

That was one of the lowest points in my life, and it still makes me sad to think of it. Not only was I being forced to leave Seattle, I wasn't even welcome in my friend's home. I felt abandoned by all parents, not just my own. I wanted to have parents who cared about me. I was so worthless, I couldn't even scrounge a little parental warmth from my friends' parents. To this day, I have a recurring dream in which I'm trying to get back to Seattle.

The rest of high school was a bust. I drank too much. I was often depressed. I was constantly trying to numb out, although I went through the motions of being an active high school student. Sarah had wanted to try a new high school when we returned from Seattle, and it had been made clear to me that my needs were not going to be met, so I don't think I even weighed in on which high school we would go to.

I didn't take any advanced placement classes, I didn't do any real college planning, and no one encouraged me to do so despite my obvious intelligence. When it was time to go to college, I just went where Sarah had gone; I was too insecure to go away alone somewhere.

Ironically, Sarah didn't even want me to go to her college. She was territorial about her friends and embarrassed by me. I was fat now. I weighed about 180 pounds.

At college, I went on a diet and exercised with my dorm mates. I jumped rope and tried to limit my food intake. Yet, when I was visiting Sarah's off-campus apartment, the conversation went like this:

"I'm doing great with my diet."

"Right," Sarah said with skepticism.

"I am! I've been jumping rope, and..."

"Well, I talked to Rusty, and he said he saw you in the cafeteria — and your tray was full."

Sarah couldn't stand me at this point in my life. When I talk about this now, I often say I don't blame her. I was pretty pathetic. The truth is, though, her words were like acid. They burned — and they left scars.

In my early college years, I came to the realization that not only was Dad different from the man he had been when he was married to Mom, he wasn't ever going to be the same again. I really began to miss the old Dad at that point. I listened to "Landslide" by Fleetwood Mac and cried.

As the damage caused by my parents' divorce sunk in, I got angry and began a few years of escape through drinking, drugs, and travel. I remember being emotionally moved by "Time for Me to Fly" by REO Speedwagon, "Needle and the Damage Done" by Neil Young, and "Running with the Devil" by Van Halen. I moved back to Seattle briefly but was so screwed up I couldn't settle in there and feel good about it. I flew to Hawaii and lived with a friend from Seattle who had married a soldier. I slept in a closet, smoked a lot of pakalolo, and came home even more pale than when I had left.

Drink, drink, drink. Cry, cry, cry. Self-pity, sob, woe. Then I got sober. I finally decided I wanted to live a decent life. And I knew no one would be interested in marrying me if I kept on the way I was going.

I didn't tell my mother I was going to check myself into a rehab program. She had tried to talk me out of treatment in the past, saying I wasn't that bad and could quit on my own, and I feared she'd try to talk me out of it again if I told her. I wonder if the thought of having an alcoholic daughter made her feel uncomfortable with her own drinking. Or perhaps she felt I was not like her father, who was a horribly abusive alcoholic, and she didn't want me to have that label. I don't know.

I remember sitting in my bedroom watching Johnny Carson and writing in my journal. Here's the entry I wrote on that night in 1983 (I was very drunk at the time):

2 November 83

Dear Johnny (Mr. Carson),

I am watching your show tonight and am thrilled with your idea to "go to bed" with four members of your audience.

You have always been a special person to me. Beyond your comedy and your spontaneity, I enjoy your humanness most. I have great respect for you.

A few years ago, I was attending Virginia Commonwealth University, and one of the girls in my dormitory was an absolute fanatic about your show. I'll admit I had never seen your show before that time. But once I saw it, I was hooked.

Karen (my dorm mate) and I got into an argument one day about the American dream. We took government class together, as well as literature and media classes. She said that people never really get what they want in life — if in fact they were even capable of knowing what they wanted. I, on the other hand, argued that one of the special things about our great country is that we can be and do what we want, if we want it badly enough. I then argued that if I really wanted to — I could even be on the *Tonight Show Starring Johnny Carson*. To this day — six years later — I still believe anything is possible.

The problem was that all these years I've never quite hit upon what I could do to impress you and earn an appearance on your show. Well — I am now an alcoholic. I guess I always have been — but two days from now I am going into the hospital to sober up and get on with my life.

Mr. Carson, if I get straight, I will shine brighter than any star you've ever interviewed. And I know that even that is not enough to get the chance to meet you. But many drinkers watch your show. You have kept me company on many a lonely and sad night. Johnny, I am only twenty-four years old. I want to be a writer and hope some day to share my experiences through that vehicle. But you can help too! If one person came on your show to talk about this sensitive and devastating problem, it could save someone's life. I want to be that person. I have a strong sense of humor, and I would be an upbeat and positive guest. Do you believe in the American dream? For many of us, you are. I know you know sadness. You are human. Will you give me the chance to reach others?

Katie

Getting sober was by far the hardest thing I've ever done, but no more difficult than long-term success with WLS. Getting sober was day after day of learning new ways to think and live. I plan to apply those lessons to my WLS recovery. I know my sobriety training will serve me well.

When I got sober, I fell in love with the songs "Time after Time," "I Can See Clearly Now," and "Shower the People You Love with Love."

I notice I don't listen to music very much anymore. I find that it makes me too emotional and brings up the old feelings of loss and trauma. The strong emotions of my youth almost consumed me, and as a mother and wife, I don't have the luxury of descending into the depths of my emotions, which have never been fully resolved. Now, I have to keep a tight rein on my emotionality, my intensity, or I can't function at all. Maybe that's one of food's roles in my life, stuffing feelings so that I don't get carried away by them.

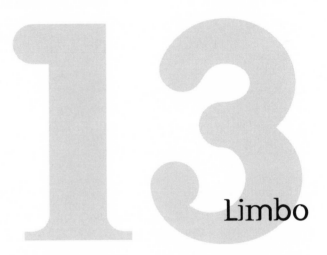

Limbo

feel like my surgery date will never arrive. It's somewhat common to have to wait a while once you've decided to have WLS. Sometimes you have to wait for insurance approval; sometimes the insurance company holds out hoops to jump through; and sometimes, like in my case, the surgeon is busy enough that you have to schedule the surgery months in advance. At this point, I'm six weeks out and I'm even more paralyzed than usual.

This morning, my husband is doing the dishes we have let pile up in the sink all week long. He works full-time, and I am an at-home mom, yet I couldn't bring myself to do the dishes this past week. I'm so darn quirky, preoccupied, and physically uncomfortable that I'm not particularly functional.

I do the bare minimum. For example, while Barrett is in school for this couple of months, I make sure he does his homework at night. I get him up in the morning, pack his lunch, and drive him to school, but even those few tasks are hard for me to do. The other day I forgot to pick him up. The school called to remind me.

My husband has begun to talk about how difficult it is to have a disabled wife. I think he has been more honest about that lately because I have been discussing my weight openly with him. He actually knows how much I weigh, which is sad and embarrassing for me.

I am always tired because I have stayed up late the night before watching TV. I just can't seem to stop watching. I hope this changes, and I get more energy once I have the surgery. I know some of my negative behavior stems from emotional problems rather than weight problems. I wonder how I'm going to overcome my emotional quirkiness after the surgery. I can't imagine being any different.

I know I am deeply entrenched in my behavioral and emotional patterns. I have been the size I am now for years. I just don't do much of anything anymore. And it all seems like so much effort, I don't *want* to do anything. What if that doesn't change when I lose weight?

When I read the online journals of people who've had the surgery, they all say how much they enjoy being active again. Will I?

My weight has been a convenient way for me to avoid the challenges of life. I have avoided failure and crushed hopes by not even trying. I haven't had to deal with the issues in my marriage that have always needed to be addressed, because I have shut down to some degree.

I just don't know anymore what is caused by my weight and what is going on emotionally to cause my weight. Obesity is a physical disease, but to be honest, for me there is a substantial emotional component. And I have to address it. The surgery won't cure what's wrong in my head, and I don't want to sabotage my future success.

Right now it's so hard to imagine being different. It's hard to imagine being energetic, vibrant, and motivated. Those words don't describe me today, and they haven't described me for some time.

My lack of entry into life is absurd, at times, and yet I still don't seem to do what I need to do. My husband just peeked in to ask if we have any toilet paper in the house.

"I'm going to run up to the store. This no-toilet-paper-thing is getting silly," he grinned at me. I'm thinking what a good sense of humor he has. He hasn't showered yet, he's in the middle of doing the chores I should have done this week, and suddenly he has to — well, you know — and the poor man doesn't even have toilet paper to use.

I have virtually stopped going to the grocery store. I can count the number of times I've gone to the grocery store this year on two hands — and it's June! We're out of napkins; there are no tissues upstairs; our paper towels are gone.

"You could use some leaves," I joke. He actually laughs good-naturedly.

"Oh, wait!" I exclaim. "There's a box of tissues in here." I'm in my office downstairs. "You don't have to run out to the store right this minute." I grin and hand him the box, knowing he's going to the grocery store for me this afternoon after he mows the lawn. I haven't considered doing yard work for ten years.

I'm not totally worthless. I take care of Barrett. I usually homeschool him; I even take him on field trips. Last year, I packed us up and helped move us to this house, which has been a great success. I feed the cats.

But I could do so much more and Mike and I both know it. But then, so could he.

Mike and I both have trouble being present in our relationship. In some ways, my gaining weight has been a way to draw Mike into our family more. He was a workaholic early in our marriage, then he went to graduate school. He resists being controlled, which is good, but he can't be pushed into anything if it doesn't meet his strict criteria for what is worth his time and energy.

Early in our relationship, I was very romantic. I dressed up for him, surprised him, took risks with him, and tried to engage him in our life. He loved how I gave to him. The problem is, he set boundaries, refused to be pushed into anything, consistently gave less than I asked for, and was rarely willing to nurture me.

I admit it. I am extremely deprived in the nurturing department. My parents were not nurturers. I long for Mike to fill that void, even knowing he won't make up for what I missed. Still, I want him to develop some nurturing skills that are appropriate in a marriage relationship. The heavier I am, the more he has to take care of me, which is a sick way for me to get some nurturing, for me to feel like I'm worth his time.

Mike, who has never been great at planning and doing romantic things for me, has become less and less romantic over the years. Not less cuddling, just less romance — flowers, surprise getaways, candles, and massages. As he has become less romantic, I have shut down. Why bother trying to inject our relationship with extra romance if it's not going to be reciprocated? I don't want him to be just like I used to be and start giving as much as I did, but he has to give more than he does.

The surgery is going to change our relationship dynamics dramatically. I won't be surprised if we'll need marriage counseling.

Well, I did it. I signed up for a plus-size women's weight-loss class at my local heath club. I decided that if I wait until surgery to start getting in shape, the surgery will be harder to recover from.

I went in a couple of weeks ago to sign up. The bone-thin instructor explained the program, took my money, and then wanted to weigh me. I didn't want her to. I have been on too many diets that involve being weighed by a skinny person who doesn't understand why being weighed is embarrassing. I refused to let her weigh me. I told her I don't want to focus on my weight. I want to focus on my health. She asked if she could measure me. Okay, I let her do that. Who cares? Then I told her what I weighed — "for my records," she told me.

Today, I got busy writing and almost forgot to go to the first class. It must have been resistance. I wouldn't have forgotten if I were going to meet with a literary agent or going to the movies. No, I really didn't want to go to class. I hid in my office while Mike did chores and I typed away, oblivious to the time. Eventually, I accidentally glanced at the computer clock. Oops. It was 1:09 P.M. The class was supposed to start at one.

I haven't showered, I whined to myself. *I'm smelly. I am not over my head cold. I don't want to go.* But then I thought, *When will I ever want to go? Never. So, I might as well get going.* I took a spit bath and headed out the door. I was forty minutes late to class. I slunk in and whispered to the scrawny instructor, "I'm sick. I'm sorry."

"Get into place," she ordered, not even smiling, while pointing to a spot in the middle of the floor. I was surrounded by a bunch of tired-looking women. The weedy instructor handed me weights and told me to start marching in place. And I did.

The rest of the hour I moved from station to station with a nice woman who showed me how to do all the different exercises. I did fine. I actually surprised myself. I did just fine. I couldn't find my pulse when we were asked to do that, but I lied and said I was "in the zone." I'm sure I was.

After class, we all said our names and the wisp of an instructor handed out T-shirts. Mine was the largest they had (XL), but it won't fit me. I'm not even going to try. The featherweight instructor also directed our attention to a chart she had posted on the wall for everyone to see. It included our weights and measurements! I was stunned. She actually said, "Don't worry, I didn't put your names on the chart. I've assigned each of you a number."

How kind of her. Considering I am by far the largest woman there, I think people will be able to figure out which woman weighs more than three hundred pounds. I was so annoyed and indignant. I know I'm fat and sensitive, but really, how much more insensitive could that pipe cleaner of an instructor have been?

Oh well. I did just fine. I'm going to keep telling myself that. I did just fine.

Let's not kid ourselves. I am making mental progress but not physical. In fact, I went to the doctor today about a sinus infection, and when the nurse weighed me, I had gained five pounds. What's up with *that?*

I have not felt much like exercising. Between the sinus infection and the evil exercise instructor, I haven't gone back to the gym. I don't want to. It's too hard. That's how it feels. Too hard. I am supposed to be mustering up inner strength now and it isn't happening. I am eating lots of sugar, sitting on my big butt a lot, and spending way too much time online at the WLS message board. I feel like I'm in a holding pattern and can't get out. I hate waiting!

I wish my surgery was tomorrow. I still have lots to do to prepare, however. I need to get all the junk food out of my house and buy protein drinks, a mini blender, and foods that are easy for new WLSers to eat. I need to rent a power recliner, so that I don't have to struggle to get in and out of bed early on after surgery. I need to see a lawyer and make out a will, power of attorney, etc. I have a lot to do. So why do I sit at my computer all day?

14

What It Takes to Change

just had an intense discussion with my husband about what it's like to have an eating disorder that developed, in part, due to the criticism I have endured in my life. During our conversation, I found myself weeping like I haven't in a long time.

After the conversation, I grabbed my chocolate pinwheel cookies from the top of the refrigerator and came downstairs to write. I won't have the crutch of cookies much longer. I plan to give up sweets after surgery.

My intense emotional outpouring began when Mike and I were chatting at breakfast. I mentioned that I wanted to get a new hairstyle. I have kept my hair long because Mike prefers long hair and it's easy to take care of. Love those ponytails!

When I brought up the potential haircut, Mike immediately launched into his opinion of a haircut I got years ago, which at first I didn't even remember getting. It was short. Apparently, really short. And Mike said it looked awful on me.

"I felt beautiful in it," I muttered, finally remembering.

"Believe me, it was awful," Mike countered.

"Some people didn't think so," I defended.

Needing to be right, Mike stated, "Charlie said it was awful too." (Charlie is my brother-in-law.)

Anger bubbled up inside me, and then I was awash with sadness.

As I began to sob, I realized how ashamed I am of how I look. Not just of the fat, but of me in general. I am ashamed of my bushy eyebrows, my small eyes, a little bump on the edge of my left ear, my chubby fingers, the mole on my face, my less-than-white teeth, my varicose veins, my upper arms, my occasional pimples in various places, the hair that grows in my armpits, my small nail beds on my little toes, and my cracked heels.

There was a time in my life near the end of my drinking, when I could not bear the thought of anyone looking at me at all. I remember working at a hotel the summer before I quit drinking, and I lived about a mile from it. I was depressed. Despondent, really, and I couldn't think of what to do for the forty-five minutes before I would have to leave for work. I had planned to drive to work as usual, but as I stood in my apartment wearing my Holiday Inn uniform, I decided I might as well walk to work. At least that would give me something to do.

I literally trudged to work with my shoulders sagging and my head down. At one point, I became aware that people were behind me and I actually began to chant quietly but audibly, "Don't look at me. Don't look at me. Don't look at me." My face burned with shame.

The walk wasn't filling the whole forty-five minutes I needed to kill, so I wandered in to the Lums restaurant a few blocks from the hotel. Remember Lums? I sat down and ordered a Tab. I sipped despondently, head still hanging low, and in short order I finished the drink. I continued to sit there, having no place to be for another half-hour. I was thinking about my dad leaving, my indiscretions with men, how ugly I was. My self-loathing came at me full force.

When my waitress set a fresh Tab in front of me, she said in a motherly tone, "Here, honey. I don't know what's wrong with you, but it looks like you could use this."

That waitress is one of the main people who inspired me to get sober. In that single act, she made me feel worthy. She didn't see the despicable me; she saw the hurting me.

People just aren't like that very often in life, especially not to obese people. And that small kindness fueled my spirit.

I needed to make changes in my life. I needed professional help, and I needed healing. I needed to feel safe and loved and valued. I needed all that supportive power, so that I could have the energy to change.

Change, the kind of change I needed to make then, takes a tremendous amount of energy and focus. When people look at an addict (food, drugs, alcohol — it doesn't matter), they often judge and wonder, sometimes out loud, why the addict has such little willpower.

But that idea is only a popular myth. Some of the addicts I have met have more willpower than their critics will ever have. We've practiced a lot. We've dieted, we've self-monitored, we've tried and tried again — often with no support. No positive energy from the outside world. I signed up for a commercial diet program, and they took my "before" picture and started me on a diet. I followed it for four months flawlessly. I liked it. I planned every meal. I exercised exactly as much as I was told to. I rearranged my life in every way necessary. Really, it was an amazing effort — and all this while my mother and others continued to tell me I was fat and disgusting.

The strength I drew on came from within. I didn't have God, because I didn't even realize faith was an option. (I was raised in an agnostic family.) So there I was — working, working, working, pushing, trying. After four months, I began to struggle. I was partying too much and losing my self-control more frequently. I held my head high, though, and continued to participate in the program.

One week, instead of losing another pound or two, I had gained a couple of pounds. No big deal. "Stick with your food plan, Katie. You can burn those two pounds off with extra exercise." Extra exercise? It was only two pounds. Couldn't I have just stuck with the program I had been given in the first place? NO. I needed to punish myself and make the hard work even more challenging. *I see you're failing, Katie. So, here's an extra burden to carry.*

The next week I had lost nothing, which was a step in the right direction because I hadn't gained anything either. But, despite my embarrassment and frustration with myself, I went back to be weighed and measured — because, silly me, I thought I was paying for the support. This time, the nutritionist flipped to the front of my chart and used her staple remover to get out my "before" picture. She held it so I could see it, and she shook it at me.

"See this? Do you want to look like *this* again?" She had an angry, disgusted look on her face.

Needless to say, I never went back.

Now, my husband, who merely wanted me to avoid an ugly haircut, felt appropriately sorry for hitting my shame nerve. He said, "This is going to be that kind of summer. We have to be prepared for the fact that your feelings are going to come up and you won't be able to use food to cope with them."

My, my. He has learned so much in husband school over the past fifteen years.

You probably think I've been sitting here writing *and* munching on the yummy, marshmallowy, chocolaty cookies I brought down-stairs with me to my office today. Surprisingly, I'm not. They're still sitting next to me untouched — a security blanket in case I need relief.

Food is one of my deepest comforts, one of my purest joys. I guess food has to be somewhat pleasurable, or else we would all starve to death. If eating were not pleasurable, the human race would be extinct. Some of us get a false idea about food early on in our lives though. It happens when we're given a lollipop after skinning our knees. Or when we have a big success and celebrate by going out for ice cream.

I have fond memories of my mother taking me to Howard Johnson's after I appeared in a play at the local community theater. The mom who taught me how to loathe myself also taught me how to soothe myself. When we had meatloaf for dinner — one of the ultimate comfort foods in our family — she would always make a half-sandwich of meatloaf later in the evening because the dinner had been so good she wanted to keep eating. Mom cut her baked potatoes in half, scooped out the soft white fluff, and slathered butter on. Then she put dollops of butter in the potato skins, along with salt and pepper, and let them sit and get melty for an end-of-the-meal treat. Mom bought snack cakes and chips. These are my fond childhood memories.

The not-so-nice memories involve the emotional detachment in my home. My father's brooding distance, my mother's endless conversations on the telephone while smoking cigarettes, Sarah's insistence that I not speak to her friends. Even the pets were a disappointment.

When I was in family-of-origin therapy (the therapy in which you learn to blame your dysfunctional family for everything bad in your life), we did a family drawing. We were adults, but we sat in a circle on the floor, paper and crayons in front of us, and drew pictures of scenes from our childhoods.

In my picture, Dad was not there. I drew the house we lived in during my elementary school years. Through the window, I showed Mom sitting at the kitchen table (smoking a cigarette and talking on the phone). Sarah wasn't in the picture either. Then I found myself drawing all the pets we had during my childhood that we had gotten rid of for one reason or another. After I drew a pet, I would take the black crayon and draw a big X over the animal.

The front yard had Domino, our Dalmatian; Misty, our German shepherd; and Chocolate Sundae, our collie. I crossed out all of them.

What happened to Domino should give some perspective on the pet situation at our house. Domino was high strung and beautiful. He had spots on his side that pushed together to form a heart. I loved that. Sadly, Domino had a problem with peeing on our drapes — our expensive drapes. At the time, I really didn't see what all the fuss was about, especially considering how friendly and fun Domino was.

Apparently, my parents didn't agree with my assessment. I came home one day to find Domino gone. No good-bye. My mom told me my dad was angry at the dog and was tired of the pee problem, so he took Domino to the pound. I was crushed. To add insult to injury, Domino's picture later appeared in the *Alexandria Gazette*. I imagine the caption said something like, "Save this sweet dog from being put to sleep. Adopt him today." I don't know what happened to Domino. I just know I lost him and it hurt. I wouldn't have been so traumatized if I had been told ahead of time and if I had not seen the advertisement. I kept imagining Domino being put to sleep, and it made me heartsick for a long time. This is one of my worst childhood memories.

In my picture, I also included the crocuses spread randomly throughout our yard. These pretty flowers sprang up every spring like a surprise, even after we moved away. I guess that was a symbol of Dad, who had allowed me to select the spots where we planted the crocuses. He had imagined putting them together in a small patch, but when I suggested putting them all over the front yard, he agreed. This is one of my best childhood memories.

I also drew in (and crossed out) Gypsy and Peachy, two cats we had lost.

What was striking to me about the experience of drawing the picture was that I did not feel at all connected to my mom, who I imagined was oblivious to me.

Hold on... I need to take a bite of one of these pinwheels.

15

It's Official: I Told Barrett

Sarah told her kids that I'm having WLS, so then I had to tell Barrett — so his cousins wouldn't tell him first! I guess that means I'm really going to have the surgery. I know I've been saying all along I am going to do it, but in the back of my mind I have been allowing for the possibility of changing my mind. I know I still can, but it's harder if Barrett and everyone around me know I have scheduled the surgery. Barrett is an old soul in many ways.

Anyway, I decided to tell him in the car on the way to school this morning, because eye contact and serious conversations during which he's supposed to really pay attention are really difficult for him. I told him that my gall bladder was not working and the doctor said it needed to come out, so at the same time I was going to have a procedure on my stomach that would make it easier for me to lose weight.

He said, "Great! That will go great with your exercise!" He doesn't know I've been balking at the exercise because of the crappy exercise instructor. I guess I better get off my you-know-what and start exercising at home.

I told Barrett about how fast the weight loss would be, and he said, "I've only seen you small in pictures. This is going to be a big change. Are you going to be able to eat sugar?" I told him about the side effects of sugar after surgery and that I was thinking I would give it up. He added, "That's great. Then it won't be around the house, and I won't eat so much either. But Dad and I can still go out for ice cream, can't we?"

"Sure."

"And you can come with us and keep us company!"

"I don't know. Mama is going to miss eating some things for awhile. I may not want to come with you."

"Oh, I get it," he said. "Well, it will get easier, Mama."

"I know. It's going to be difficult at times. You may see me cry a little bit from time to time, but our lives are going to be so much better. It's really worth it."

"I can't wait to go swimming with you. Can you go to the creek with me after you feel better?"

"I'd love that," I said.

Barrett exclaimed, "I'm glad you're doing it this summer. I can take care of you!"

"You can, but you'll be out playing and going to summer camp. I plan to get my friends to help too. And, of course, Daddy will help a lot."

"I bet it will be hard for a while," he said.

"Yeah, I hope it's not too hard. I'm really going to work at taking care of myself."

"Oh, don't worry, Mama. Now do you want me to tell you a joke that will make you feel better?"

"Sure."

"Well, Garfield is chasing Odie and Odie runs away and climbs a tree. Then Garfield says, 'I guess it's easier to do something you can't do when you don't know you can't do it!'"

I chuckled.

"Do you get it, Mama? You'll do it, even if right now you don't know that you can do it."

I'm embarrassed to admit it, but I have never made a will. I'm sure a lot of people don't have a will, but now that I am about to go under the knife, I figure I better do it. We met with the attorney yesterday.

Now I am filling out a long form that is asking what I want to happen to my property when I die. Of course, most of it will go to my husband and son. I also want to leave something to Sarah, my niece, and my nephew. The girls are easy — jewelry. My nephew, however, is more of a challenge. I can't imagine what I have that he would want.

I have been wandering around the house looking at all my possessions, trying to figure out what to leave my nephew. The lump in my throat hurts. I love my life. I love my family. I don't want to die. Imagining Barrett's life without me is almost too painful to bear.

What can I leave my nephew that I would not want Barrett to have? Ah ha! I just noticed a wooden incense box on the shelf in my office. That will work. It's beautiful, and he could keep it on his desk or dresser.

When I was a kid, I went to see the play *You Can't Take It with You.* I don't want to take anything with me when I go. I just don't want to go.

This coming week, I am going to the hospital to have all my pre-op testing done. The only test I'm nervous about is the arterial blood gas test. I overheard someone saying the test involves sticking a needle into an artery. Ouch. I hope that's the extent of the yucky stuff. I know the surgery is much more extreme, but I plan to sleep through that part of this ordeal.

During the early part of recovery, protein drinks are an essential part of the diet, as is water. So, I tasted a protein drink a couple of days ago. I found it to be tolerable, albeit a bit too sweet. I am going to try a few brands before surgery, so that I'll have some sense of where to start once I get home from the hospital. During the first couple of months I will also be allowed pureed foods. The key is to have moist things I don't have to chew. After a couple of months, I'll begin to eat regular food but will have to take very small bites and chew thoroughly.

All the pureeing and chewing are necessary because the passageway from my stomach into my intestines will be about the width of a pencil. I'll even have to crush my medications, which should be tasty — not!

I'll have a much more stringent vitamin/mineral regimen after surgery. Because part of my intestine will be bypassed, I won't be able to absorb as many nutrients from what I eat. If I don't supplement with vitamins and minerals for the rest of my life, I will suffer malnutrition with potentially dire consequences. I plan to buy what I need this week and start taking the stuff now. My surgeon's nutritionist said it's helpful to get used to the regimen before the stress of surgery.

I also need to rent a recliner so that I don't have to get into and out of bed for the first week or so. I'm going to buy some DVD sets of old TV shows. I want to distract myself as much as possible after surgery in case I have a lot of head hunger.

Based on how sad I've been feeling the past few days, I am worried I will miss food and go into a depression. That may sound strange, but when I really think about the roles food plays in my life, I know I will have a big mental adjustment to make. I won't make it all at once, I know. It takes time to get used to a new way of life. I also will have to get used to watching others eat and to preparing food for others. I expect it will be quite tough at times.

Some of my new WLS cyber friends tell me to stay positive. They suggest working on letting go of negative thoughts. That is a tall order. I am the quintessential negative person. I ricochet between laughing about the absurdities of my situation and crying in self-pity for the burdens I've carried.

I am terrified I will sink into depression after surgery. When I had Barrett by emergency cesarean, I got very depressed. I'm sure some of it was hormones related to pregnancy and birth, but I also worry that some of it was caused by the anesthesia.

Deep down, I am still a drug and alcohol addict. The thought of being drugged during and after surgery scares me — partly because I crave that feeling of being drugged. Of course, that's part of the reason why I overeat. I've always felt the need to suppress part of myself. Substance abuse, including my sugar addiction, has played a role in my coping abilities for almost my entire life. I want to think that I will be so different after surgery that I will not want to self-medicate, but as I have heard said over and over again, *gastric bypass isn't brain surgery.*

Unfortunately, my stinkin' thinkin' will not be removed along with my gall bladder. My disordered thinking got its start years ago. My friend Karen has been asking lately, "What is the lie that you believed when you were hurt as a child?" I remember feeling like I wanted my parents' attention, but I knew they were not going to give it to me — not enough of it, anyway. I don't know if I was needier than some kids or if my parents were more distant than some parents. Maybe both. I know my own son is very demanding. He is vibrant and full of ideas, and he wants to interact all the time. I have paid a lot of attention to him over the years, in part because I didn't want him to feel marginalized the way I did. Karen believes that evil comes into our hearts and minds when we are emotionally vulnerable. When we experience traumatic events as children, they cause us pain and invite lies into our mind. Those lies then define the choices we make throughout life. One lie I integrated into my being at a very young age was: *I am not worth anyone's time.* Others were *I am too much,* and *I overwhelm people.*

As an adult, I was diagnosed with ADHD. That might explain my feeling of being "too much" for everyone when I was a child. I also found out I have a rather high IQ — another reason I might have been "too much." But the lies tell me I will always be too much for anyone I meet and I will always be more needy than a normal person.

Intellectually, I know I'm not "too much," but I haven't been able to let go of the lie. To avoid being too much for people to handle, I have dampened my energy with depressants, most recently sugar. I don't allow myself to fully be myself. That is why it has taken me so long to start publishing — to start working in the field I feel passionate about. I have to learn to counter the lies with the truth — there is plenty of room in the world for my sometimes excessive personality.

Because I feel too needy, I have never allowed myself to ask for what I want. I have become a master at asking for what I think you want me to need in the amounts I think you are able to give.

I have never had a natural sense of what is okay to ask for. We have cultural norms, of course. And I have used them to limit myself. If I might be too much, then I must not ever ask for what I really need, and *God forbid* I ask for more than my share. I don't even know what my share is anyway.

16

Finding Peace

I had completely forgotten, or had never known, how much like my father I was until I went to visit him a couple of times when my stepmother was dying of brain cancer. During one of my visits, Dad and I watched the Clinton-Lewinsky debacle unfold on the *Today Show*. Dad gave a running commentary about what was happening and what he thought about it. I learned a lot about his political and social values and I was stunned at how similarly we felt. I then realized how deeply he was ingrained in me. I remember feeling so much peace and validation when I realized that.

Dad taught me how to paint during one of those visits. He had taken up oil painting a few years earlier and offered to stand beside me while we each painted the same mountain landscape, with him instructing me along the way. That painting I did with my father hangs in my house now, a symbol of our evolving relationship and my love for him. I love that he is always learning something new, even now.

I know Mike loves me unconditionally, because he took one look at the painting I did with Dad and hung it in our bedroom where he could look at it all the time. Honestly, it's not a very good painting, but Mike says it reminds him of how talented I am.

Similarly, my stepmother loved my father unconditionally, and she probably loved all of his paintings. Early in Dad's painting career, he created a particularly unpleasant painting, according to him, and of course she loved it. In fact, she insisted they hang it on the wall. Dad obliged her, hanging the painting in their bedroom over the door so that no one could see it when they looked in, but she could see it when she was in bed.

When my stepmother died, Dad wanted to select some meaningful items to place with her in her casket. We walked around their apartment and discussed what might be appropriate. Of course, Dad wanted her singing medals to be placed around her neck. She had a beautiful voice and sang often. That is one of my fondest memories of my stepmother.

When we wandered into their bedroom, the painting over the doorway caught Dad's eye.

"I never did like this painting, but she loved it," he remarked. Then he retrieved it from the wall. It was small enough to fit at her feet in the casket, he pointed out. Dad and I delivered the items to the funeral home, specifically telling them to put the painting at her feet.

I don't want to minimize what a hard time this must have been for my father. His second wife had been the light of his life. He had cared for her through years of cancer, and now she was gone. Yet, amazingly, my father kept his sense of humor.

We attended a service at the Catholic church the evening before the actual funeral. The casket was to be placed at the front of the church so that mourners could see her one last time. Dad and I sat in the front pew, watching the funeral-home employee set up the area where the casket was situated. The casket sat on a wheeled cart, and a curtain drape hid the cart. It seemed everything was ready for the viewing when the funeral guy squatted down, parted the curtain, and retrieved Dad's painting and an easel. He then set up the easel at the head of the casket and placed the painting on it in full view.

I was in shock. Dad was quite surprised too, but he kept his wits about him. He leaned toward me and whispered, "Don't worry. They'll think she painted it."

This week, I went to the hospital for my nurse interview and pre-op testing. The test I was most worried about was the arterial blood gas test — the one I'd heard horror stories of pain and suffering about. Luckily, it was the very first test I had, and my nurse had delicate, almost magical, hands. I hardly felt the needle at all. She said some technicians try to rush, and that is what usually causes the dreaded pain. Well, she took her time, and I was quite grateful.

Much to my distress, I am beginning to get anxious about the possible pain and humiliation that often go along with impersonal healthcare settings. I've tried to stay upbeat about this whole process, but even during my pre-op tests, my fight-or-flight system took over. I was shaking slightly and my mouth was dry.

My pre-op nurse said she has had gastric bypass surgery. I was relieved to have a nurse who understood some of what I'm going through. She was a knockout, though, and I suspected she either didn't start out as heavy as I am, or she had had plastic surgery to remove all the sagging skin. Bingo! She was much smaller than me when she had the surgery — at least seventy-five pounds smaller.

She said to wait for two years before deciding about plastic surgery. She said I am young enough that my skin might shrink more than I expect. Also, she encouraged me to get enough protein, water, and vitamins. She suggested exercise, including lifting weights, once I have completely healed from the surgery.

The nurse claimed her food addiction did not come back with a vengeance after the surgery. That was exciting to hear, but I still don't believe that will be the case with me. I have read numerous accounts of people having trouble following the guidelines for eating after surgery. Maybe the online message boards I'm reading are not a representative sample though. Maybe the people who are the most successful don't turn to the message boards for support as often as those who struggle. Who knows? I go to the message boards because I'm an information addict and an extrovert.

The nurse added to my long list of things to buy. At first, all medications and vitamins will need to be chewable, liquid, or dissolvable under the tongue. Also, I won't be able to take any extended-release medicines after surgery.

I finally reserved my power recliner this week, but I still need to buy some DVD sets for entertainment. (We don't have cable upstairs where I'll be recuperating.) I bought several Tupperware products, including various shaker/mixers, two-ounce storage containers, and a couple of large *SpongeBob, SquarePants* cups with lids. I didn't see a grown-up version of cups with lids; otherwise, I would have bought the *Judging Amy* cups or the *West Wing* cups.

Barrett is jealous of my SpongeBob cups, so I've already agreed, under duress, to share them with him, which means they're his now.

Sarah and I have hired a sitter to help us this summer while I am indisposed. Under normal circumstances, I would have shared the driving to the various camps we're sending our kids to, but after surgery I won't be able to drive for a couple of weeks. I feel relieved we have hired support.

Apparently, I'll need to arrange for other support as well. A woman's bra can irritate an incision line, so I will have to come up with an alternative. I'll need *something*. A friend suggested I just wear a camisole under the big abdominal "wrapper" in which I will be sent home from the hospital. (The abdominal support is necessary to keep me comfortable and to help prevent a hernia.) A camisole won't be enough support for me, but I'm going to buy one, just in case I can't figure out anything else.

After surgery, I won't have gastro-esophageal reflux disease or heartburn. My blood sugar will be stable and low. I won't have upward-creeping blood pressure. I won't have so many aches and pains. It won't hurt to bend over and pick something up off the ground or to lean in to eat a meal. I won't get winded walking to the bathroom. The seatbelt buckle in the car won't dig into my side. I won't be a slave to sugar. I won't feel so awkward and exposed when someone makes a fat joke (although I'll still be offended).

I won't have to squeeze into restaurant booths, friends' cars, airplane seats, chairs, lines, carnival rides, bathtubs, or shoes. I will be able to sleep on my stomach again. I won't be too embarrassed to get my hair cut or to get a pedicure. I will be able to shave my legs with ease. I won't snore. My asthma will get better. I'll have better eating habits, which means Barrett will have better eating habits. I'll be able to ride a bike. I will not have to avoid activities that involve standing up for long periods of time. I will be able to grocery shop comfortably. I will be able to wear regular-size gowns at the doctor's office. I won't dread being weighed by the nurse. People won't look the other way when I pass by. I won't avoid new experiences out of fear of being judged for my fatness. I won't put off my goals and dreams, thinking people won't take a fat person seriously.

Other than knowing Mike will be happy that I can resume household chores, I don't know what he won't miss. More honestly, I don't want to think about what he won't miss because I feel so guilty that he has to put up with my disabilities. I don't think I'll ask what he won't miss — I don't want to encourage him to spend time thinking about what he doesn't like about me and our situation. After all, what if I change back someday and he has admitted how much he hated me the old way? I think that it's unlikely he *hates* me the way I am, but I know I make life harder for him.

Barrett is looking forward to being active with me. He is used to having a sedentary mother who is in pain most of the time. (I try to be as cheerful and active as I can be despite my limitations, but I am pretty limited at this point.) Barrett wants to go on long walks with me, go swimming together, ride bikes, go hiking, and on and on. He won't miss me saying, "I have to sit down. You go..." And he won't miss being my errand boy in the house. He is forever fetching something for me (as is my husband), and while I still intend to order them around as much as I can get away with, I'll actually be capable of doing things for myself.

Although he doesn't know how to articulate it, Barrett probably won't miss my apathy. He wants me to do what I love to do and of course he wants to help.

I took him out to lunch after basketball camp today. During the ride to the restaurant, he asked me what I was doing while he was at camp.

I told him, "I'm working on my book."

"Your mystery novel!" he exclaimed.

"No. This is something different. I am writing about my life. I am writing an autobiography that discusses my life-long struggle with my weight and talks about my upcoming surgery."

"That's great! Am I in it?" His excitement was palpable.

"Yes, you're in it."

"Is my name in it?"

"If you want it to be."

"I want you to mention my name! What have you said about me?"

I tried to remember what I had said about him so far. "Mostly, I tell stories about you that also have something to do with the main topic of the book. Like, I included the talk we had when I told you I was having the surgery."

"Oh, okay. You can tell people I love bunnies and that orange is my favorite color. Well, before that it was red. You can tell the whole story about what colors I like, if you want."

"Okay, sweetie, I will," I reassured him.

"It will be so different when you're... you're..." he hesitated.

"Skinny," I filled in for him.

"I'm glad you'll still be able to eat at restaurants with Daddy and me. Even if you do just have a little bit of Daddy's dinner."

"I'll still be able to eat almost everything once I heal from the surgery."

"Good. Everything but sugar, right?"

"That's right, love bug." I didn't mention the refined foods and snacking I'd be skipping after surgery.

Even though Barrett won't miss my sugar-zombie ways, I think he will miss having sugar in the house. That's probably the only thing he will miss.

The Countdown Is On

It's hard to believe I'm only three weeks away from WLS. Someone told me the last few weeks before surgery would speed by and she was right. In addition to finalizing my revocable living trust, I have been ferrying Barrett back and forth from day camp, and I'm going from store to store looking for the various vitamins and foods I'll need after surgery.

All I really want to do is zone out. I want to eat the things I love (that have been lovingly prepared for me by someone else, using groceries purchased by someone else) while watching my favorite shows on TV with my feet up, uninterrupted. I don't want to be driving from here to there in the car, dealing with strangers. For instance, when I'm around my new attorney, I feel embarrassed about my need for a haircut, my lack of makeup, my rotundness, and my sleepy face. I am so tired.

I feel frustrated that I can't shut down and travel inward. That is how I prepare for big, emotional traumas, as this surgery is bound to be. I don't want to be a wife or a mommy for a little while, and that's precisely what is so hard about being a wife and mommy. You know, no days off.

I am almost looking forward to the couple of weeks after surgery when I won't be able to drive — it will sure limit the errands.

I called and reserved a recliner two weeks ago — trying to be efficient. Well, the rental place still hasn't guaranteed one for me. They keep saying, "We have one being repaired, but we're not sure it will be ready in time. Call back in a few days." Finally, today I began to call around to other furniture rental stores, and no one has a power recliner. I am so frustrated. Ever since I heard the idea, I have been obsessing about renting one. A regular recliner won't work as well, because without the power, you have to strain your stomach muscles to get the footrest down.

My house is a wreck, because my husband brought my computer up from the basement office so I won't have to walk a lot of stairs early on. To set up the computer, we displaced a lot of other stuff. Now I have to put that stuff away.

Also, we are reorganizing our kitchen to accommodate all my new supplies and equipment. I bought a mini blender to puree my food and mix my protein drinks. I bought a slew of vitamins and minerals. I got that big Tupperware order. I have begun to buy condiments and protein powders.

I also bought tongs at Kmart yesterday. Martha Stewart's were particularly interesting, because they curve at the end in a way that makes them seem like they'll be easy to adapt for help with personal hygiene. Yes, there are some rather unpleasant aspects to this. I won't be able to bend to clean myself, so I'll use the tongs to hold the toilet paper or washcloth. I can't bring myself to practice this, but I really should. I don't want to have to learn everything right after I've had major surgery.

I have been taking smaller bites of my meals and am practicing chewing everything to death.

Mostly, I'm just paranoid that I'll get sick and have to postpone the surgery. I have a headache and some sinus symptoms. Barrett was just diagnosed with strep.

I don't want my surgery postponed, but I feel a sad resignation about the foods I am giving up, especially the chocolate bars with almonds and the chocolate peanut butter ice cream. I know I'll get used to the new way of eating, but I worry.

I read the journal of a woman who lost more than two hundred pounds after WLS. In her journal, she listed the types of food she was eating and I was shocked. She was eating unhealthy foods. Will I do that? I sure hope not. I don't want to just lose weight. I want to be healthier. It's hard to imagine getting healthier while eating a lot of canned spaghetti, fast-food sandwiches, and fries, while drinking massive amounts of diet soda. I don't mean to be judgmental; the woman is thrilled with her weight loss.

The truth is, however, I can understand this. I am a food addict. I can't imagine enjoying eating normally. I don't even know what that is. I will never get to a place where I can trust my choices with food "in the moment." If I follow my lifelong pattern, I will *always* want more.

The weight regain that is happening to some longer-term WLS recipients is scary. I am terrified I will regain my weight, which makes me feel determined to be hyper vigilant about the necessary lifestyle changes. There are some people having this surgery who either have not been well-informed or who have a great deal of denial about the need for lifelong weight management following WLS.

I just think it's a slippery slope back to the old eating habits. That's how it would be for me, and that's exactly what I want to avoid.

18

The Aftermath

Well, I survived. The first week or so after surgery was rough — pain, nausea, and gas took turns causing me a lot of irritation — but I am finally feeling a bit better and have gotten some perspective.

I tried to write in the hospital after surgery, but the morphine blocked my wits. I did write a bulleted list the day after surgery. I wanted to make sure my account of the experience included all essential information. Here is my list:

- Deb
- clear liquid
- fever

- me
- pigtails

Intriguing, isn't it? Deb was my roommate, and she was great. I guess I was having a clear liquid diet. I ran a slight fever for a couple of days, because I was not able to breathe deeply and cough. (Therefore, I was awakened at all hours to have nebulizer treatments.) I don't know why I put "me" on the list, but it *was* all about me. And the pigtails? That's how I wore my hair. I didn't care how I looked. I was all about function. I was sleeping on my back, and the ponytail hurt.

My surgeon was great. I have had no complications to date. Everyone who saw my incision at the hospital complimented me about how good it looked.

At the same time, the hospital's staff was hit or miss — and sometimes horrible.

When I woke up from the surgery, I felt pretty unsettled. I was in pain and nauseous, but they kept giving me medication until I was comfortable. It's a blur now, all except hearing the woman next to me, who was in great distress, call for help when she felt like she needed to throw up.

The nurse yelled across the room to her in a gruff voice, "Then throw up!"

I couldn't believe how harsh the nurse sounded. The poor, nauseous woman turned out to be my roommate, Deb. Deb also had WLS, and she shared the semi-private room with me for the duration. I loved that! She and I took turns harassing the aides, a couple of whom were horrendous (some of whom were exceptional). They barged in and out all day and night, slamming things, talking loudly, and giving us bad advice like, "Measure your pee," and then, "Don't measure your pee; you don't need to," and then, "Why didn't you measure your pee?"

I know now that it would have been better for me to have an advocate at the hospital. Even the best hospitals can be bad in any given moment. The first day it took them four hours to find the time to take me to the bathroom — I'm not exaggerating!

My aide refused to help me in and out of bed on the afternoon of my surgery, saying, "You have to learn how to do that yourself."

Nice. I was sore and still a bit disoriented. I wish I had a video of getting back into bed by myself after my long-awaited first pee. Although getting out of bed was tough, getting back in was even tougher. Over the course of three days, I developed an elaborate method to get in bed.

Stand with my back to the bed. Get up on wobbly tiptoes, lift buttocks, and sit as far into the bed as my short legs would put me. Then hoist, lean, roll, flop, scooch, push a random bed adjustment button, scooch, flop, give up, pass out. It was pathetic! It wasn't until *my last night* in the hospital that a kind aide finally showed me how the bed railing came down and told me how to get in with ease.

My clear-liquid (that is, my protein-spiked Jello) breakfast was two hours late the first two mornings, which seemed odd to me considering I had had major gastric surgery and required a special diet and appropriate timing. My surgeon's assistant told me I should not drink anything for thirty minutes before a meal, but the thirty minutes turned into an hour, and I was miserable. Then, despite my late breakfast, the nurses wanted me to eat lunch the minute it arrived.

My stomach was now the size of a thumb, but apparently no one had educated the hospital staff about that. Right after I dutifully ate lunch, the nurses insisted I take all my medications together crushed up in a cup.

Needless to say, I was nauseous and miserable for a couple of days. After the second late breakfast, I started refusing to eat if they didn't bring a meal at the right time. That was freeing.

My third day, pureed food was served. The smelly fare was served in the center of a large, dull white, scratched, cafeteria dinner plate — a small brown puddle and a small green puddle. Mmmm. My roommate asked me (the morning of our last day there) what I had learned that was helpful during my hospital stay.

I replied, based on the previous evening's meal, "I learned that I do not like cat food." Deb and I were laughing so hard that we had to hold our pillows on our tummies and close the curtain between our beds so we wouldn't look at each other and provoke more painful laughing. Bottom line — my surgeon did an excellent job. But if I had it to do over, I'd make sure I had someone to stay with me in the hospital who knew how to push the staff for good and safe care.

I am home now, following all the instructions rigorously, and I feel relatively good (now that I have control of my environment).

I wish I had gotten ahold of an incentive spirometer before surgery and started doing some deep breathing. Even blowing up balloons would have helped. I wish I had done that. I ran a low-grade fever at the hospital because I needed to be able to take deeper breaths and cough up stuff. Luckily, I didn't get pneumonia.

To take the nasty crushed pills, I have resorted to using lite whipped topping. I coat the bottom of the teaspoon with it, sprinkle on the crushed pills, and use another teaspoon to put a thin layer of whipped topping on top of the medications. A small sandwich. The medicines are reasonably tolerable that way.

I feel so bummed out sometimes, despite my new lease on life and the good reasons I had for having the surgery. I just said good-bye to Mike and Barrett. They are going out for dinner at Red Robin and are planning to visit the mall, neither of which I feel up to at the moment. Having four tablespoons of a restaurant meal doesn't sound good to me (it's just a tease!), and because it's the end of the day, I'm a bit worn out. So here I sit alone. To make matters worse, our phone is out for some reason, so I can't call a friend or get online with my support group. So I write. Writing is not what I want to be doing now. I want to be eating french fries dipped in ketchup.

Despite my blue mood, I consider today yet another good day. Successful. Barrett and I went for a walk. I can actually walk around the big block in our neighborhood now. We moved into our house two years ago, and until today I had never done that.

Barrett is a great walking companion. We have had the nicest talks lately and our walk was no exception. He was so excited about our trip around the block, he high-fived me and we both laughed with happiness. That's why I had the surgery. I must remember that when I get sad about french fries.

The WLS life is regimented. I pay attention to what I'm putting in my mouth (or not putting in my mouth) every waking minute. I drink sixty-four ounces of water every day, and I take six different vitamin/mineral supplements at prescribed intervals throughout the day. I drink two protein shakes and eat three small meals. My food at each meal consists of two tablespoons of pureed protein and two tablespoons of pureed fruits or vegetables. I may not drink for thirty minutes before or after my meals. And then there's my whipped topping-coated medications.

I started walking when I got home from the hospital. My doctor wanted me to start with ten minutes a day and increase my walking time by three minutes each week. I'm up to about twenty minutes a day.

I get better at the routine every day. I can't imagine having to start back at a job at this stage of my recovery, although most people do. I am giving myself time for a gentle recovery.

It's hard watching my husband eat. When he cooks a meal, it's a big production, and for the first week or so, I got mad at him every time he cooked. In the evenings, I even let him know it. I was tired by that time and just didn't keep it together emotionally as well by nightfall.

While the "head hunger" is hard, I get full pretty quickly when I eat my little meals. If I don't feel full, I can usually chalk it up to wanting to eat, not to being truly hungry. I don't miss sugar at all. Can you believe it? Maybe this will change, but I really think I've turned a corner. I'm getting a small taste of feeling better and I don't want to go back.

Even when I walk, I can feel a difference. My stomach isn't as heavy, so my back doesn't hurt when I walk. And that's at three weeks. I can only imagine how energetic I'll be in three months! I don't know how much weight I've lost. I'm just not going to obsess about the scale, but I did measure my waist this morning, and I'm two inches smaller around the middle. I thought my pants felt a tad looser and, by golly, they were.

I've tried to eek out as much time as possible in my rented recliner, but sadly the rental place came to pick it up today. I have slept in it for nearly a month. I have to admit, I'm not excited about sleeping in my bed. Even though it's been almost four weeks, I feel discomfort in the area of my incision, and I can't imagine being comfortable.

Being in the recliner in the middle of the living room between the TV and my computer made me feel safe. The overstuffed blue chair was my security blanket. After returning from the hospital, I sat in it when I felt tired or upset or was in need of comfort. I held the little brown bear, Snicklefritz, Mike and Barrett had brought to me in the hospital. I called him my "coughing bear," because he was the perfect soft thing to hug when I needed to sneeze, cough, or laugh. (Laughing still hurts!)

I cried like a baby when they came to pick up the recliner. Mike suggested I rent it for another month, but deep down I know it's time to move on.

I know once I'm in my bedroom again, I'll remember all the things I love about it — the hum of the ceiling fan, the quietness, no cats to bother me in the night, and MIKE. It will be nice to sleep next to Mike again.

19

Travels and Travails

During my second post-op month, I went on my first road trip. I was picking up Barrett, who had been visiting his grandparents, and we met at a restaurant to do the kid swap. I couldn't eat anything on the menu at that point, being on pureed foods for my first six weeks. It seemed like most of the food on the menu was fried. Much to my surprise, I handled the situation with relative ease. I didn't feel really jealous of what everyone was eating. I ordered a decaf coffee and sipped it slowly. I was so relieved I didn't crave what others were having. Maybe my head hunger was going to go away. What a relief. The main awkwardness I felt was worrying about whether or not my in-laws thought I was weird for not eating, but I knew I couldn't let that get to me. I just acted like everything was normal and tried to minimize any discussion of my surgery.

When I look back at my early WLS days, I expect I'll treasure my memories of walking with my friend Julia most of all. Julia has become one of my biggest supporters. I don't know what I would do without her. I met Julia in a neighborhood Bible study group. She and I were both working at losing weight. We realized we shared a love of writing, and that is how our relationship really began. Julia shared her science fiction writing with me, I shared this manuscript with her, and we went on long walks and talked about our writing and our lives.

What I like about our walks is we didn't say, "Let's walk three times a week," or "Let's walk Mondays and Wednesdays." We walk every evening when we are home and available. I like that better than the quota system. It makes me feel like I'm walking because I want to, not because I have to. Subtle, but it makes a difference to my rebellious heart. The message I seem to internalize from our arrangement is that my default setting always is to walk with Julia. All things being equal, we're walking. I like the ebb and flow of it. I like that I can cancel on a busy evening and know that Julia and I will walk again as soon as we can. I like knowing that Julia believes I am committed even when I have to cancel. She never shames me or wags her finger. And I never do that to her. It's simply lovely.

At first I thought walking at 8 P.M. was not good enough. (I am still a self-critical soul, no matter how much I fight that in myself.) I have heard on more than one occasion that exercise first thing in the morning is the best for women, because it gets the metabolism going. Well, I wasn't able to exercise first thing. Okay, I didn't want to. Besides, walking in the evening during the hot months of summer helped me avoid sweating. I hate sweating.

The lesson I have learned from this experience is that any exercise is better than no exercise. My weight loss is excellent. I feel good, look good, and have hope. Could my weight loss be even better if I exercised in the morning? Maybe. Who knows? But is my exercise regimen fun and working well? Absolutely. Am I losing enough weight? Yes! Am I thrilled? I am beginning to feel real joy about all this. Real joy.

And it's not just my walks with Julia that thrill me. Barrett and I have been taking long walks to the post office and the store. It still pains me to think of all the opportunities I missed to be active with Barrett over the years, but we're making up for it. We pack our little insulated, backpack lunch boxes with water and whatever else we need (I usually need to bring a protein supplement with me). We bird watch along the way. I am always amazed to see how far we can go.

Okay, I admit it. There is one small problem with the walking. I have foot pain. I was sure it would go away once my weight came down, but that's not happening. So I went and got X-rays of my feet. We'll soon see what's going on.

I have always loved road trips, and my first long trip after surgery involved traveling to Charlotte, North Carolina, to see my great aunt (actually, Mike's great aunt). Barrett and I stayed in a hotel so that I could have complete control of my food. I find it harder to visit people and have them cook for me when I really can't eat a lot of what they fix. I don't eat breads, pastas (unless they're whole grain — and even then I don't like how they taste anymore), or desserts. I have to drink my protein supplements and take vitamins. I just like having a safe haven when I'm traveling.

The problem with the trip, though, was that I had to eat at restaurants a lot, and over time, I've found that too much restaurant eating gets my food cravings stirred up. One evening I had ordered meatloaf, mashed potatoes, and green beans to go. (Remember, I was still at the four-tablespoons-of-food-per-meal stage.) In my hotel room, I found I couldn't stop eating when I was supposed to. I'd had my quarter cup or so and was feeling full, but I just wanted a few more bites. It tasted too damn good — not in a healthy way but in a comfort-food way.

I remember thinking, "Damn it, I don't care if I throw up. I'm going to eat a couple more bites." That's a scary place to be. It felt like the old, sick me coming out to haunt.

Thankfully, I didn't throw up the few extra bites I took, but I did get a stomachache and knew I wouldn't be repeating that behavior again for a while. The cool thing is that I realized I made a mistake and decided to not do that again — and I haven't. Somehow, it feels like the surgery has given me a lot more control of my eating. I notice an old behavior in myself that I know won't serve me well anymore, and I make a decision to stop it. And I can. That just blows me away.

Episodes like the meatloaf debacle remind me I am still a food addict. I know not all obese people are, but I know down to my bones that I am.

By the time I was three months post-op, I was down sixty pounds. I still looked and felt fat, and I was still wearing some of my size twenty-six clothes — but that didn't bother me very much. I had lost enough that I knew the surgery was working for me. And I was trying to be good with my food, water, supplements, and vitamins, so I knew WLS would keep working for me. I had worn stretchy clothes for years, so I have to assume I was bigger than size twenty-six when I had the surgery.

Now that some time has passed, I've discovered four things I hate. First, I hate people noticing my weight loss and using that as a cue to evaluate out loud their own weight and diet issues. I'm sorry, I don't want to "talk diet." I especially hate being a reminder to others that they need to change their eating habits!

Second, I hate telling people I've had WLS. What a hot button! People are really opinionated about it and don't hesitate to tell me why it's wrong to do it.

One friend said, "I know a good nutritionist," in response to my musings about wanting to find a good one. She added, "But she doesn't believe in weight loss surgery, so I don't think she'd be a good choice."

I responded, "It's sad people are so ignorant about this surgery."

"Oh! She's not ignorant," my friend said.

Ignorant is exactly what this lady is. I realize this is a surgery of last resort. The thing is, some people get to a point where a last resort is necessary. Sometimes it's the most humane course to follow.

In my case, I was on the brink of becoming insulin dependent. All of my previous diets had been unsuccessful and I wanted to live a better life. Just surviving every day was a chore.

After WLS, I went home from the hospital already off three diabetes medications, and my blood sugars are the lowest they've
been in years. My pouch keeps me from reverting back to old
behavior. I have a window of opportunity to make lifestyle changes
and to learn how to deal with the myriad challenges associated
with WLS and weight loss.

Third, I hate head hunger. Head hunger is the hunger you
think you feel even when your body is not hungry, and it's the pits.
I get it when Mike is eating a particularly aromatic, high-fat, or
high-carb meal. I get it when I have strong feelings about almost
anything. And I think I get it during a certain time of the month,
although I haven't pinned that down yet.

Sometimes I go for days with the constant desire to snack.
Mostly, I resist. The main difference between this feeling of head
hunger and the deprivation I used to feel on diets is — and this
amazes me — I don't feel extremely deprived. I tell myself to
acknowledge the longing and move on. Although I have feelings
of loss daily, I don't let myself wallow in them. I tell myself sternly,
"Katie, you chose this. It's your ticket to the life you've always
wanted." That really seems to help me. Self-pity just brings me
down. If I pass a food counter stacked with sweets at the store, I
feel loss, disgust at my eating disorder, and disappointment
momentarily, but then I feel resignation and move on. It's not fun.
But it's not excruciating either.

I make sure that I love the meals I make for myself. I don't settle for meals that are just so-so. I think that makes a big
difference.

In a few months, I'll begin to feel more real hunger. I will have
to religiously use this tool I've been given. I'll eat only at meal-
times and won't graze and snack to sabotage my WLS journey. I

won't drink high-calorie beverages. I just won't. The journey to this place has been too hard. I won't let it be for nothing.

Fourth, I hate plateaus. Plateaus drive more WLS patients crazy than almost anything. I hit a plateau that lasted for two weeks recently. My support group leader told me that this is normal. She told me to go home and measure myself. Wouldn't you know it; I had lost several inches even though the scale hadn't moved. I still wanted the scale to be moving down faster, but I knew I was really doing just fine.

The scale can make you crazy. Many dieters, including me, use the scale to determine how they feel about themselves on a given day. In the past, when I noticed the scale sticking or moving up, I almost always threw in the towel and started eating what I liked. Clearly, the diet wasn't working, so I might as well eat.

I've learned now that it doesn't pay to obsess too much about my weight. I don't allow myself to weigh in every day. It's not motivating to me. I have gone through WLS to be comfortable, healthy, and productive. I know I need to be thinner to reach my goals, so I want that too, but I don't have any illusions that I am going to be some tight-skinned, sixteen-year-old beauty queen.

My healthier attitude about the scale tells me I am finally ready to close this self-destructive chapter in my life for good and change my relationship with food. I know I can't afford to go back to my old behaviors. But it's still scary. People still struggle with food after surgery. For some, at first it's trying to find things they can tolerate and that taste good. For others, it's battling the head hunger. Many people don't feel hunger at all for a long time. Eventually, though, we all get hungry again.

I actually experienced some physical hunger early on, and I'm grateful for that. I feel relieved that I won't be magically not hungry for six months to a year and then suddenly feel it. By having a little real hunger now, I can practice how to handle it. When the hunger comes back in full force, it won't be a shock.

I try to stop at the first sign of satisfaction now. I hate that! I miss stuffing myself. I just don't miss how sick that made me feel. For me, a full pouch does not feel the same as a full stomach. Sometimes I long to stuff a big bite of something in my mouth, like a sub, but I know it won't feel good once it's swallowed.

I've heard it said many times now: WLS is stomach surgery, not brain surgery. Dealing with my emotional and psychological issues will be a crucial part of my success. This new way of life is a learning process. I will always have opportunities to learn to use the many tools available to avoid unhealthy eating and battle head hunger. I am grateful for my little pouch, especially. That's the best tool of all.

20 Finding My Future

decided to go to a publishing convention to learn what I needed to know to publish this book I'm writing. It's embarrassing, because I'm obese and writing a book on weight loss surgery. I had to muster up a lot of courage to introduce myself and say why I was there. People were polite to me. No one openly criticized me or my goals.

I am amazed that I already have a strong vision for myself. I was in prison and now I've been set free. I have so much to do, so much lost time to make up for. It's exciting to be a person who has big plans! Before, I was resigned to never being the productive person I could have been if only I weren't so huge. Now, I feel an obligation to do the things I had almost written off.

Sometimes we lose weight and say, "Now what?" Or we lose weight and realize our weight wasn't our only problem. We discover psychological problems, behaviors that hurt us, and feelings we had been successfully stuffing down with food. Our relationships change, our needs change, our wants change. Metamorphosis can be stressful!

I only feel the stress, because I can do just one person's work, when in reality I have enough goals for a dozen people. My hope is that I resolved a lot of my psychological issues, identified my self-destructive tendencies, and grappled with my fear of success the last several times I lost weight. After all, I've done the therapy and support groups for years. I'm hoping that my major issues won't be tripping me up because I've worked through them already. Only time will tell. In the meantime, I'm going to act as if I'm a healthy person. It can't hurt.

While I was at the publishing conference, I took time to drive to the suburbs and visit one of my dearest friends, Pat. When I visited Pat, I was really worried that she would be angry with me — or hurt — because I didn't tell her I was going to have weight loss surgery. She had never been the kind of friend to get hurt easily, but I didn't know the limits of her tolerance for and acceptance of me and my situation.

I made the drive out to her home with butterflies in my stomach, but the minute I walked in the door and she gave me a hug, I knew I had been worrying for nothing. Silly me. I so easily forget when someone loves me. I guess that has to do with all the years of confusion about my parents' love.

I told Pat all about my WLS, and she accepted my choice with sensitivity and good humor. I was so relieved and instantly reminded why I have valued her friendship so much over the years.

Pat and her family traveled to our house for Thanksgiving the following month. I'm not one to cook huge meals for housefuls of people. I have never aspired to be a gourmet cook. So I didn't feel compelled to make a huge variety of delectables. And no WLS patient should. I figure I'm trying to recover from a life-threatening disease, and I don't have to put myself in difficult situations that could lead to poor choices. I planned what I felt comfortable with and served it to everyone. Pat brought a pie, and I had made sugar-free pudding for myself as a treat.

I ate slowly, sipping decaf the whole time, so that I could eat just a little more than normal. I know. I'm not supposed to do that, but I have only done it that one time and it was so worth it. After the dinner, I didn't feel very satisfied. I was full, but I wanted to eat more just for the experience of it. It was the aromas, textures, and temperatures. The pure joy of eating. That is one thing I miss from time to time, being able to have some more.

The only way I could think of to solve this dilemma was to have Thanksgiving leftovers for breakfast, lunch, and dinner for the next three days. That worked for me. In the end, I felt like I'd had my share.

Three memorable things happened at my first post-op Thanksgiving. First, Pat and I went for a walk together, and I was thrilled to be able to do that with her after my embarrassment at Disney. Second, when I opened the turkey to prepare it for cooking, we realized it was spoiled. Pew. So, we sent Mike and Pat's husband to the store for another turkey.

Alas, all they could find were a small ham and a chicken. That was our Thanksgiving dinner. Pat and I laughed our way through getting the meat into the oven and making the side dishes. We laughed even harder, though, when we realized we had gotten so busy talking we forgot to put the side dishes in the oven. We wound up cooking the mashed potato casserole at five hundred degrees to make sure everything would be done at the same time.

Third, I was not overly focused on eating. I enjoyed the food, but I enjoyed the company more. I didn't obsess about anything and I had a blast.

I went to a candle party last night. I am allergic to many scents, so it was silly of me to go in the first place, but my walking buddy was giving the party and I wanted to support her. I didn't think to bring food with me, though, and that was a mistake. My friend had been kind enough to make a sugar-free dessert and served that alongside some tantalizing baked goods. I didn't happen to care for the sugar-free dessert and wasn't sure I wanted to get into any sort of sweets habit — even sugar free. It was hard to be around the eating and drinking of sweet stuff. I wish this wasn't an American custom, but it is. At least it wasn't a cookie exchange party. Cookie exchanges are deadly for me. In my former life, I always wound up taking a variety of cookies home and then eating them all myself. Not good.

At the candle party, I wanted to eat in general more than I wanted the sweets. I am happy about that. Craving sweets would be the pits. It's hard enough having head hunger. That's what gets stirred up at social events like this. I just get too excited about the food. I start to obsess about it. I can't imagine I'll ever enjoy parties the way I used to. Once you eliminate the alcohol, sweets, and snack foods, what's left? Chatting with people who are eating cocktail wieners dipped in barbecue sauce just doesn't do it for me. Jealousy sets in.

I admit it. I was getting a bit of an ego over the fact that I hadn't ever barfed after surgery. It's not that uncommon to throw up. Usually, it occurs when a food isn't chewed well enough and gets stuck where the pouch empties into the intestines. For five months, I was a model of perfection, first pureeing everything I ate, and then chewing oh-so-thoroughly as my diet progressed to solid food.

New Year's Eve ended my perfect record, however. I had decided to allow myself a few hors d'oeuvres, but I must not have been chewing carefully, or perhaps the snacks were too high in fat — I'm not sure. All I know is that I was running down the hall to get sick and wondering why I had let that happen. Oh well. Experiences like this just give me more resolve to do the right thing — to take care of myself and be responsible for my choices.

Parties are hard. I'll keep working on it.

21

Super Kitten

I **was so excited** as I approached the six-month post-op mark that I began weighing myself daily, which I hadn't been doing during my WLS recovery. I had been weighing maybe once a week. As I began to weigh daily, I realized I was getting awfully close to a hundred-pound weight loss. I kept telling Mike and Julia I knew there was no way I could hit the hundred-pound loss by my six-month anniversary. I felt disappointed, but I knew I couldn't.

Much to my surprise, a few days before the anniversary, the scale registered a bigger than normal drop. I was two pounds away from my interim goal. At exactly six months post-op, I was exactly one hundred pounds down! I had my six-month appointment with the WLS surgeon and couldn't wait to get there. I felt so proud.

As soon as they weighed me at the office, though, I realized my scale had been wrong. Home scales just can't be trusted. I hadn't lost 100 pounds — I had lost 110!

Mike got some time off work, and we decided to take a family vacation at Disney. Mike had not been able to go last year when I met Pat there, so now we wanted to see Florida together. At first, I was excited about the trip, because I wanted to do Disney on foot. No wheelchair for me! Sadly, that desire was soon squashed. My foot pain, which still had not cleared up, suddenly got much worse.

I was afraid to go to the foot doctor, because I was worried about being shamed for my weight. (Technically, I am still obese). I made an appointment and then cancelled it, then I rescheduled it. I was so nervous. Finally, I had my appointment. There was no scolding from the foot doctor. I found out that I needed orthotics, because my foot was being injured when I walked. Apparently, I walk on the outsides of my feet. I didn't even know I did that. The bad thing is my orthotics won't be in before we go to Disney. The foot doctor said to use a wheelchair. Now, that's irony.

What a difference a year makes, though. With Pat, I spent my trip wanting to sit in the wheelchair as much as possible without seeming lazy. With Mike, I spent the trip being annoyed because he was making me sit down so much. I ached to get walking. Wow. So, I didn't do Disney on foot, but I wanted to. *I wanted to.*

Barrett and I shared one great accomplishment on this second trip to Florida. On our first trip, I had let Barrett climb the stairs of an historic lighthouse with strangers because I could not make the trek myself. This time, Barrett and I climbed to the top of the lighthouse together. What a joy!

Someone once said, "The only exercise some people get is jumping to conclusions, running down their friends, side-stepping responsibility, and pushing their luck." That was me. I hated exercise. No, I hated to hurt and sweat. I still hate it, but now that I'm healthier, exercise doesn't hurt quite as much. I guess I'll just have to accept the sweating, dang it.

I may get infections this summer under my skin folds. I look like a Shar Pei dog at this point. My boobs are at my beltline, and my lower stomach reaches below my pubic area. Not thrilling. Actually, it's kind of embarrassing. Mike and I joke about it, and I know I have to accept this new body. Hating it won't make me happy. The only choice I have is to do the best I can with what I've got. (Besides, I look great in my clothes.)

I joined a new gym. I've always liked this gym, and I knew I would never go back to Slim, the personal trainer. The man who signed me up at the club introduced me to a trainer who was especially sensitive and responsive to her clients. I knew I liked her when I told her I didn't want to do something and she said, "Okay."

What a relief. No guilt trip. She didn't judge me. She just started with me where I was — emotional baggage and all. She understands I have to feel physically *and* emotionally safe to get invested in working out. She understands resistance and works to keep me focused on my goals. I just love her.

I'm working with a nutritionist now too, and I don't feel nearly as resistant as I used to. I am trying so hard to follow her suggestions. I feel much less shame when I show her what I've been eating. I get tired of feeling so embarrassed about what I eat, especially when it's what I'm supposed to be eating.

I am squirreled away right now at a local all-suites hotel to write. It is hard to write at home with all the distractions and I wanted a big block of time to think, stew, meditate, and ponder. I brought all my own food this time, thus solving my restaurant/hotel/food dilemma. I crave other food, but I am at peace with bringing my own. In fact, I feel great about making this healthy choice for myself.

Yet, here I am in the midst of success and still feeling guilty about how I think and feel about food. I feel guilty that I am craving something salty. If I were at home, would I have resisted the craving? I pray that I am not at the tail end of a pink-cloud recovery from WLS. Many people I've talked to say it gets tougher to make good choices further out from surgery. I know what that feels like. I've gotten there with every diet I've ever been on.

So far, whenever I start to get even slightly off track, I immediately miss the healthy, planned eating. The stakes are so high I seem to finally have accepted how costly it is to give in to temptation. I know my inner obese self (the 200-pound gorilla) still waits to be let out again. I must keep her locked away. I cannot give her even a teaspoon of leeway. If I don't handle the end of the pink-cloud stage differently from the way I've handled this stage on past diets, I am doomed to repeat my mistakes.

Mike is amazed at how functional I am these days. I'm spry, I'm sexy, and I'm energetic. (And I can cross my legs, fit in restaurant booths, and eat with a plate in my lap — I actually have a lap now!) I know Mike loves the changes. He is relieved to have help around the house. And I love how he is supporting me by expressing concerns while not being a mother hen. He spent so many years watching me self-destruct, I'm sure he fears a relapse on my part. I try to reassure him.

A couple of days ago, I started recording again what I eat and when I take my vitamins and supplements. For the first three months post-op, I recorded this stuff every single day. While I am doing fine now, I've noticed some old habits trying to creep in. Nothing drastic. Just a handful of popcorn here, an unmeasured meal there. I don't like the feeling of pushing the limits anymore. That is always how I return to failure. So, I am recording again.

One night, I left my record sheet on the kitchen table when I went to bed. The next morning, I noticed Mike had drawn a cartoon on the sheet. It was a picture of a kitten (me) wearing a cape, standing with arms akimbo, the initials *SK* on her chest. *Super Kitten*, I mused. The still, small part of me that knows she will succeed feels like Super Kitten, although I don't admit it to anyone.

That little cartoon is a great example of how Mike shows support — not by picking at me so much as by praising me when I do the right things. It's awesome.

And I am doing the right things. Here at the hotel I have been working out on the treadmill, writing, and following my regimen. Never in the past have I used free time like this to be self-nurturing and productive. Usually, alone time like this would be used for overeating/binging, feeling sorry for myself, and trying to figure out what the hell is wrong with me — all while watching endless TV. Not this time.

Dr. Phil often says past behavior predicts future behavior. So, I am amassing successful experiences now, hoping they will rewrite my future — a future in which I get to live out my dreams with the people I love, a future that is not dictated by my obesity and illness but rather by my compassion, sense of humor, strength, and love.

I think about obese people feeling hopeless, and it just breaks my heart. I know WLS is not for everyone, but for some of us it's the most humane ticket out of an imprisoned life. When I think about all the other types of surgery people have for far less critical reasons, I am confused by the sensationalism and negative opinions about WLS. Why are we so heartless toward obese people who are suffering? Would we divulge all treatment options, including the one with the best potential outcome, to a cancer patient? Of course we would.

I wish there were better options than WLS. I wish diets didn't have such poor outcomes. I wish our society would clean up its food supply and stop marketing crap that hooks people and then slowly kills them. I wish I hadn't inherited genetics that predisposed me to obesity.

Mostly, I wish people who are suffering with obesity would have the courage to demand better care from the medical community. My gastroenterologist, who was treating me for acid reflux caused by obesity, had almost no knowledge about WLS. He did not offer it as an option at any point in our conversations. When I finally asked for information on the subject from him, he printed it off the Internet and gave it to me. Gee, thanks. Did he learn to use the Internet in medical school? I'm great at the Internet. Maybe I could be a doctor too.

No matter how thin I become, I will always be obese. I see people larger than me now (what a change), and I know that on the inside I am just like them. I pray I will always be vigilant, because I will always love food. I am human.

Once, in a guided imagery session during group therapy, I was taken on a journey to find myself as a small child. I remember my quest vividly. I boarded a golden sailboat, which sliced through a blue-gold ocean, heading toward a rising sun. I was on the bow, leaning into the wind, absorbing its power. My hair fluttered behind me. I felt confident. When the sun was fully up, the boat landed on a beach near chalky cliffs, and I jumped down and ran toward a dense conifer forest that lined the beach. As I pushed through the trees, slender branches brushed my face. The ground was soft and smelled of autumn. I noticed I was getting younger and smaller with every step.

I enjoyed the sensation of getting smaller. It seemed the smaller I got, the happier I was. I was not only feeling confident now, but I was giddy and powerful and clear-minded. I saw a cabin in a clearing. The cabin was white and had a long front porch with rocking chairs lined up on it. I stepped inside the front door, knowing later on I'd be back outside to rock. I passed comfortable, sunny rooms with flowered upholstery and ceiling fans that hummed happily.

Finally, I breezed into a study lined with floor-to-ceiling book-shelves. I was a toddler now. I scanned the rows of lovely books. I couldn't read their titles, but I longed to. I noticed a book with no title on a shelf almost too high to reach. I stood on tiptoe, stretching my arms as high as I could, and pulled at the bottom corner of the book, which fell heavily into my hands. This was the unwritten book of my life and I was overjoyed at the thought of filling it. My small eyes squinted into a smile. I knew great things were in store for me.

What I discovered from that guided-imagery session was how I felt in my life until I was about two years old. I lost that hopeful little girl awfully early.

I've noticed, lately, I feel like that golden child again. Like my life is a great book waiting to be written. I am still complicated, but for me, the world is full of possibilities. And for the first time in many, many years, I feel unimaginable joy.

Photographs

I have included just a few photos of my life. One of me as a child when I was five, and three photos that give you a sense of how my weight loss progressed after surgery. I went from wheelchair bound, an observer of life, to an enthusiastic participant! (Of course I made sure to include my guys: Mike and Barrett.)

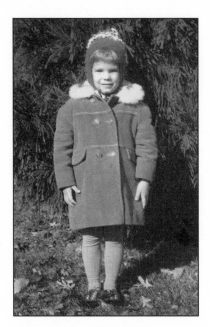

Me on my first day of Kindergarten

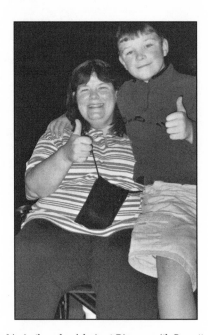

Me in the wheelchair at Disney, with Barrett

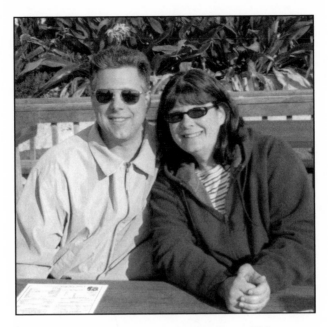

Mike and I in Florida, six months after my WLS

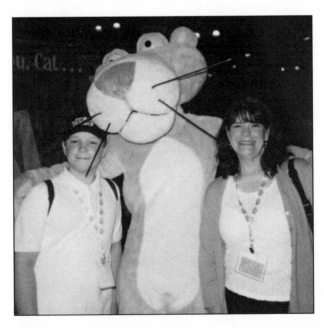

Barrett and I at a book conference, on the first anniversary of my WLS

Discussion Questions

ying to Change is an ideal selection for weight loss surgery support groups and book clubs, and it promises a lively discussion.

In her story, Katie Jay raises issues, reveals strategies, and talks honestly about life as an obese woman. She also shares her musings about why her particular genetics, upbringing, and life experiences led her to the pain and sickness of obesity, as she grapples with how to create a successful future.

The following questions are intended to stimulate discussion and allow group members to compare and contrast their experiences with Katie's — all with the goal of understanding the obesity mindset and taking personal responsibility for their own life transformation.

1. The author, Katie Jay, begins *Dying to Change* with a description of how she dealt with her food problems while her mother lived with her and with a vignette from her trip to Disney World with a friend. What do you immediately learn about Katie? What information can you glean about her personality and her character?

2. Katie clearly has strong feelings about the way her parents handled her weight and food choices. How were weight and food issues dealt with in your family?

3. Katie describes her mother as being disgusted by fat. How do you think her mother's attitude about fat influenced Katie?

4. Katie uses food to deal with strong emotions. She worries about her son's emotional connection to food. Does emotional eating get passed on to children? If so, how?

5. What is Mike's role in Katie's life? What do you learn about his character and personality?

6. The divorce of Katie's parents has played a major role in Katie's life. Discuss the effects of the divorce on Katie.

7. Katie says Barrett's school smelled like sugar. Discuss the role of sugar in children's lives and the mixed messages they receive about sugar.

8. How did Katie's father influence the way Katie behaved and related with the opposite sex before she was married?

9. How would this story have been different if it had been told from Katie's mother's point of view, from her father's point of view, and from Sarah's point of view?

10. In what ways is Katie similar to her mother? Her father? Discuss the role of addiction in Katie's family of origin.

11. How does Katie deal with grief and loss? Does she deal with it differently as she matures?

12. When the waitress at Lums gives Katie a free soda, how does that influence Katie's sense of herself? Have you done anything similar to help another person? Has anyone reached out to you like the waitress reached out to Katie?

13. Why does Barrett hate self-discipline? How do you feel about self-discipline?

14. Katie describes a rigorous lifestyle change after weight loss surgery. Do you think weight loss surgery is the easy way out?

15. How can setting good boundaries improve a weight loss surgery patient's chance for success?

16. Katie says, "Some of us, the complicated ones, have so many hurdles it seems ridiculous. What is God's purpose in *that*?" How does Katie answer that question? What might God's purpose be in allowing suffering? Do you think God causes suffering sometimes?

17. What bothers Katie about the thin exercise instructor?

18. Is obesity a choice?

19. Why do you think Katie chose Mike to be her husband? Did their relationship contribute more to Katie's obesity or to her recovery?

20. Is Katie cured from obesity? What do you think her future holds? What is the significance of Katie describing herself as the golden child?

Acknowledgments

I appreciate the help and support of many people in getting this book to press. Paula Peck read my early manuscript and encouraged me to follow my dreams. Fern Reiss (www.expertizing.com) provided wise consultation and inspired me to dream even bigger dreams. My early editors, Diane Feldman and Mariane Mears, were a great help. My substantive and final editor, Nina Taylor, did the fine-tuning this book really needed. Brian Taylor and the team at Pneuma Books contributed to this process in ways too numerous to mention. I also want to express my gratitude to Julia Persing, my walking buddy and chief kibitzer. Thanks to you all.

Thanks to my sister Sarah, who has walked beside me through everything (not a day goes by that I am not grateful for you). To my late mother, I send prayers of thanks for the many years you encouraged me to pursue my love of writing. To my father, thanks for your loving support and understanding regarding my need to tell my story, even the painful parts. Thanks to my sweet brother in NYC for giving me nothing but unconditional love.

Last but not least, thanks to Lori Sasek, Stephanie Bigelow, and Bill Wilson — you know what you did for me. And thanks to my WLS friends who have supported me on my journey to better health and fulfillment.

I am surrounded by such loving and wise people, I am truly blessed.

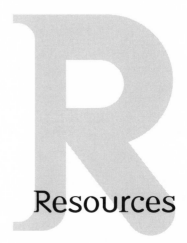

Resources

Books

Boundaries: When to Say YES, When to Say NO to Take Control of Your Life by Dr. Henry Cloud and Dr. John Townsend (From a Christian perspective, but an excellent resource for anyone!)

Boundaries with Kids by Dr. Henry Cloud and Dr. John Townsend (From a Christian perspective, but an excellent resource for anyone!)

Boundaries in Marriage by Dr. Henry Cloud and Dr. John Townsend (From a Christian perspective, but an excellent resource for anyone!)

Exodus from Obesity: The Guide to Long-Term Success after Weight Loss Surgery by Paula F. Peck

Weight Loss Surgery: Understanding and Overcoming Morbid Obesity — Life before, during, and after Surgery by Michelle Boasten

I'd Kill for a Cookie: A Simple Six-Week Plan to Conquer Stress Eating by Susan Mitchell and Catherine Christie

Weight Loss Surgery: Finding the Thin Person Hiding Inside You, Second Edition by Barbara Thompson

The Success Habits of Weight-Loss Surgery Patients by Colleen M. Cook

Weight Loss Surgery for Dummies by Marina S. Kurian, Barbara Thompson, and Brian K. Davidson

Integrating Body Self and Psychological Self: Creating a New Story in Psychoanalysis and Psychotherapy by David W. Krueger

Websites

www.edap.org — Eating Disorders Awareness and Prevention, Inc. (EDAP)

www.nawls.com — National Association for Weight Loss Surgery, an online community offering support, information, and resources

www.wlsfriends.com — an online support community

www.wlslifestyles.com — a weight loss surgery magazine

www.obesityhelp.com — an online support community (they publish a magazine too)

www.vitalady.com — a place to learn about and purchase bariatric vitamins and supplements

www.bariatricadvantage.com — bariatric vitamins and other products

www.asbs.org — American Society for Bariatric Surgery

www.fitday.com — a place to track your calories, weight loss, exercise, and more

www.bariatricsupportcenter.com — home of The Success Habits of Weight-Loss Surgery Patients™ and the International Bariatric Support Group Registry

www.thekatiejay.com

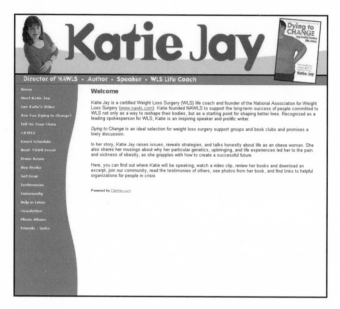

Meet Katie Jay! Visit www.thekatiejay.com to get useful information, videos, and testimonials about weight loss surgery, Katie Jay's speaking schedule, books, and more!

Free Monthly Newsletter

To receive a free monthly e-mail newsletter about maintaining success with weight loss surgery from the National Association for Weight Loss Surgery (NAWLS), e-mail katiejay@nawls.com or visit the nawls website at www.nawls.com.

Ordering Information

Pink Sky, Inc. books are available online and at
your favorite bookstore.

Quantity discounts are available to qualifying
institutions. All Pink Sky, Inc., books are available
to the booktrade and educators through all major
wholesalers.

For more information, email the publisher at
katiejay@nawls.com
or visit www.pinkskyinc.com